UNDERSTANDING AND TREATING PSYCHOGENIC VOICE DISORDER

A CBT Framework

UNDERSTANDING AND TREATING PSYCHOGENIC VOICE DISORDER

A CBT Framework

PETER BUTCHER, ANNIE ELIAS
AND LESLEY CAVALLI

John Wiley & Sons, Ltd

Other Wiley Editorial Offices

John Wiley & Sons Inc., 111 River Street, Hoboken, NJ 07030, USA

Jossey-Bass, 989 Market Street, San Francisco, CA 94103-1741, USA

Wiley-VCH Verlag GmbH, Boschstr. 12, D-69469 Weinheim, Germany

John Wiley & Sons Australia Ltd, 42 McDougall Street, Milton, Queensland 4064, Australia

John Wiley & Sons (Asia) Pte Ltd, 2 Clementi Loop #02-01, Jin Xing Distripark, Singapore 129809

John Wiley & Sons Canada Ltd, 6045 Freemont Blvd, Mississauga, ONT, L5R 4J3

Wiley also publishes its books in a variety of electronic formats. Some content that appears in print may
not be available in electronic books.

Anniversary Logo Design: Richard J. Pacifico

Library of Congress Cataloging-in-Publication Data

Butcher, Peter.
    Understanding and treating psychogenic voice disorder : a CBT framework / Peter Butcher, Annie Elias,
and Lesley Cavalli.
        p. ; cm.
    Includes bibliographical references and index.
    ISBN-13: 978-0-470-06122-0 (pbk. : alk. paper)
1. Speech disorders.   2. Voice disorders.   3. Somatoform disorders–Treatment.   4. Speech therapy.
I. Elias, Annie. II. Cavalli,   Lesley. III. Title.
[DNLM: 1. Voice Disorders–psychology.   2. Voice Disorders–therapy.   3. Cognitive Therapy.   4. Speech
Therapy.
WM 475 B983u 2007]
RF510.U5344 2007
616.85′560019–dc22   2006033490

A catalogue record for this book is available from the British Library

ISBN 13: 978-0-470-0-6122-0

Typeset in 10/12 pt. Times by Thomson Digital
Printed and bound in Great Britain by TJ International Ltd, Padstow, Cornwall
This book is printed on acid-free paper responsibly manufactured from sustainable forestry in which at least
two trees are planted for each one used for paper production.

He who is in harmony with the Tao
is like a newborn child . . .
It can scream its head off all day,
yet it never becomes hoarse,
so complete is its harmony.

Lao Tzu

CONTENTS

ABOUT THE AUTHORS

Peter Butcher BA (Hons), MPsychol, CPsychol, Associate Fellow of the British Psychological Society(AFBsPS); and an accredited member of the British Association of Behavioural and Cognitive Psychotherapies (the BABCP).

Peter has experience working as a cognitive behaviour therapist since the 1970s, a special interest in sharing psychological skills with others, and 20 years association with speech and language therapists working with psychogenic voice disorders. Peter has published widely in international journals on CBT and related subjects, including psychogenic voice, and he has presented papers on these subjects at national and international conferences.

In the field of training non-psychologists in the use of psychological methods, Peter has co-edited *Sharing Psychological Skills*, a special issue of the *British Journal of Medical Psychology* in 1985. In the area of psychogenic voice disorders, Peter has authored or co-authored a number of research and theoretical pages, as well as co-written (with Annie Elias and Ruth Raven) *Psychogenic Voice Disorder and Cognitive Behaviour Therapy* (Whurr, 1993) and co-authored (with Lesley Cavalli) a case study of combined speech and language/psychological treatment in *Wanting to Talk* (Whurr, 1998).

Lesley Cavalli MSc BSc(Hons) CertMRCSLT, Specialist Speech and Language Therapist and Lecturer in Voice, Speech and Language Therapy Department, Great Ormond Street Hospital NHS Trust & Department of Human Communication Science, University College, London.

Lesley Cavalli currently combines her clinical work at Great Ormond Street Hospital with a lectureship in Voice at University College, London. She started her career as a Speech and Language Therapist in 1988 and has specialised in voice disorders in her clinical work, teaching and research for the past 16 years. Her current clinical post involves the tertiary assessment and treatment of children and young adults with a wide range of ENT-related conditions, including psychogenic voice disorders. She is the lead Speech and Language Therapist for the Joint Paediatric Voice Clinic at Great Ormond Street Hospital and Deputy Head of the Speech and Language Therapy Service.

Annie Elias, Specialist Speech and Language Therapist in Voice, The Kent and Canterbury Hospital.

Annie Elias has worked with children and adults with voice disorders since qualifying as a speech and language therapist in 1980. In her first post at The Royal London

Hospital both Annie and her colleague Ruth Raven began working in a model of co-therapy sessions with Peter Butcher. Together they explored combining voice therapy with CBT and this led to several journal articles and an earlier text. Annie moved to Kent in 1986 to become Head of Speech and Language Therapy Services for part of East Kent. She has maintained a specialist clinical caseload in voice and is a visiting lecturer in Voice at University College, London.

FOREWORD

A human voice reflects the condition of the individual at the moment he or she speaks. It is the product of the speaker's anatomy, physiology, neurology, cultural background, health and psychological status. The synergy of these foundation elements affects the structure and function of the vocal tract and, in particular, the larynx and vocal folds. Consequently, the study of the human voice is pursued by many disciplines, both artistic and scientific, and ranging from those whose main concern is with voices which might be regarded as falling within normal limits to those which might be judged to be superior, such as those of vocal performers, or pathological, as in the case of individuals with voice disorders.

The effect of a disordered voice (dysphonia) or complete loss of voice (aphonia) is usually much greater for affected speakers than the difficulty of making themselves heard. When it is within normal limits, in addition to rendering the oral message audible, the voice conveys paralinguistic features which enhance or refute the language employed by the speaker. Equally important, listeners make judgements about the speaker according to the amalgam of acoustic parameters such as pitch, loudness, vocal quality and flexibility. Speakers who do not have the full range of vocal features and nuances at their disposal have to cope not only with the obvious practical disadvantages but also with the difficulties of conveying the subtleties of conversation and self-image which are an integral part of human interaction.

The development and increased use of videostrobolaryngoscopy, the gold standard of laryngeal examination, during the past 30 years, has resulted in the potential for much more accurate diagnoses of the causes of voice disorders. It has also resulted in the establishment of multidisciplinary voice clinics in the best centres globally. The core disciplines in such clinics are ear, nose and throat surgeons and speech and language therapists/pathologists who specialise in the analysis, diagnosis and treatment of patients with voice disorders. In some centres, members of other disciplines, such as voice scientists, psychologists, osteopaths and singing teachers also contribute their expertise. The most important task initially is that an accurate medical diagnosis of the cause of the voice disorder should be made; this is the responsibility of the ENT surgeon ultimately. Decisions are then made as to whether the treatment should be surgical, medical, a course of voice therapy or a combination of these elements.

Traditionally, a diagnosis of psychogenic voice order is a diagnosis of exclusion. It is made when thorough laryngeal examination and, where necessary, more extensive investigation does not reveal any organic cause for the voice disorder. Until now, it is at this point that terminology and classification have been vague, interchangeable and non-specific, frequently resulting in inaccurate usage. Terms such as 'functional

dysphonia' and 'conversion symptom aphonia' are used routinely to refer to psychogenic voice disorders, with little regard for their true meaning or the actual aetiology of
the condition concerned. Clinicians are also aware that in addition to being a primary
feature, psychological aspects occur in a variety of voice disorders as secondary and
compounding elements. On the basis that accurate terminology and classification is
relevant to the intervention undertaken, this book makes an important contribution by
clarifying a classification structure and by developing relevant terminology. It then
proceeds to build on this carefully considered foundation to explain, suggest and give
practical examples of the way in which cognitive behaviour therapy can be used in the
treatment of psychogenic voice disorders.

This text is unique in its careful analysis of the issues involved in both the diagnosis
and treatment of psychogenic voice disorders. It is also unusual in the field of voice
pathology in demonstrating the obvious benefits of close collaboration between speech
and language therapists/pathologists and psychologists. Through their writing here
and in previous publications, the authors demonstrate the enormous benefits which
clinicians, and therefore their patients, can derive from working in an experienced
multidisciplinary team. They acknowledge how much they learn from each other; the
result is a text in which the contributions from each discipline are recognised as being
complementary and essential. This book succeeds in making its well-considered case
for the use of cognitive behaviour therapy by speech and language therapists/pathol-
ogists as an important element of a battery of therapeutic techniques. It should enable
experienced clinicians to further develop their skills and give the less experienced
insight into the complexity of psychogenic voice disorders and their resolution. The
authors are to be congratulated on producing a thoughtful and reflective text which
clearly encompasses their combined clinical experience and their ongoing commitment to improving treatment for individuals with psychogenic voice disorders.

LESLEY MATHIESON FRCSLT
Visiting Lecturer in Voice Pathology
Institute of Laryngology and Otology
University College London
January 2007

FOREWORD

Human voice has an intimate relationship with emotions. To start with, voice can induce emotions. In adolescence, during the most emotional time of our lives, we spend considerable amount of time and resources having our emotions stirred by listening to vocalisations recorded for this simple purpose and produced by singers who, just on the strength of modulating their voice, become objects of love and admiration. But the relationship goes the other way as well and emotions affect human voice. It is the core assumption of the diagnosis of psychogenic voice disorder that emotions can actually disrupt normal functioning of the vocalisation system.

Overall, the notion that a lot of physical symptoms have a psychological origin is not as solid as it once appeared. From early psychoanalytical lists of psychogenic somatising disorders only a few remain. From skin diseases to asthma, illnesses once considered suitable for psychotherapy are now seen to be of physical origin. Not long ago, stomach ulcers were widely attributed to stress, until Warren and Marshall discovered they are caused by helicobacter pylori and curable by antibiotics. The field is plagued by the famous ease with which a neurotic conflict can be found if we only look hard enough. Psychoanalytically oriented therapists have the dubious distinction of improving the hit rate to impressive 100% by postulating that if the patient shows no neurotic symptoms or behaviour whatsoever, this by itself proves that they are converting their emotional turmoil into whatever physical disease they suffer.

As far as certain types of voice disorders are concerned though, the psychogenic hypothesis holds well. The psychological causation can be obvious, and psychological treatments evidently useful. The authors of this book are of course well aware of the dangers of over-diagnosing emotional effects, and they take care to discuss, for instance, the tricky feat of differentiating distress caused by illness from that which may be its cause. The diagnostic process is covered extensively. The book provides a thorough coverage of an important and under-served field. It discusses a range of key issues concerning the assessment and cognitive behavioural treatment of psychogenic voice disorders, accompanied by useful practical examples and case studies. Peter Butcher, who leads the team of authors, is known in the field as an experienced, sensitive and humane therapist and a versatile thinker. These characteristics are evident throughout the book. The authors have put together probably the best and most detailed resource available to learn about the practicalities of dealing with this often mysterious and disabling condition.

PETER HAJEK
Professor of Clinical Psychology
Queen Mary's School of Medicine and Dentistry
University of London

PREFACE

The genesis of this book really goes back to a day in the early 1980s. At that time both Annie Elias and Peter Butcher were working in the Out Patient Building of the London Hospital, Whitechapel; the Department of Speech and Language Therapy being on the second floor and the Department of Psychology situated a floor above. On this auspicious day, Annie approached Peter with a request. She said she had a number of 'non-organic' aphonic and dysphonic patients that were not responding to standard voice therapy or, if they did respond, they quickly relapsed. From her observations of this group of patients Annie thought there might be psychological factors making them difficult to treat. She wondered, therefore, whether Peter would be willing to see some of these patients in order to offer an opinion. Peter vividly recalls thinking and saying 'Well, I know nothing about voice disorders but the patients sound fascinating and - if there is a psychological cause - I can't think why cognitive behaviour therapy wouldn't have something to offer.'

As a result of this discussion, Annie and Peter arranged to see the patients jointly so that they could share their respective knowledge of assessment and treatment in voice and cognitive behaviour therapy. This collaboration and mutual support quickly bore fruit and their joint assessments not only revealed a variety of individual differences but, more importantly, showed interesting commonalities in the psychological characteristics and personal conflicts of these patients. As a result, this led naturally to a particular psychological focus in the treatment they began to offer. In this way, the joint sessions became an exciting journey of discovery in which the clinical psychologist became familiar with psychogenic voice disorders and the speech and language therapist had first hand contact with cognitive behavioural interviewing and treatment techniques.

Annie and Peter were particularly fortunate in being joined for parts or much of their journey by other interested and enthusiastic colleagues, including Ruth Raven, Jenny Yeatman, and Lesley Cavalli from the Department of Speech and Language Therapy at the London Hospital; David Littlejohns from the Department of Therapeutics at the London Hospital Medical College; and Catherine Austin, clinical psychology doctoral student from the University of East London. They also gained inspiration and encouragement through their contact with other specialists in the field of voice – especially Arnold Aronson in America and Janet Baker in Australia – who in their own writing and research have stressed the importance of psychological factors in medically unexplained voice disorders.

What were the findings of the initial study of 19 individuals that suggested new ways of looking at the origin, the nature and the treatment of psychogenic voice disorder?

Three things emerged. First, these cases indicated that the traditional Freudian concept of hysterical conversion - while a helpful way of viewing some individuals - did not adequately describe what was happening, psychologically, in the vast majority of patients. Secondly, the psychological assessment pointed to particular cognitive behavioural factors that were influential in triggering and maintaining the functional voice disorder in around 9 out of 10 patients. Thirdly, the new formulation suggested that cognitive behaviour therapy techniques should be of value in treating the majority of patients and, when this was explored, the approach produced very encouraging results. After reaching these (initially very tentative) conclusions, it was particularly encouraging to discover that the findings were being independently supported by other researchers using larger samples and random controlled studies.

Another implication from the research was that speech and language therapists ought to be familiar with cognitive behaviour therapy when working with voice patients and that co-therapy with an experienced therapist can be an ideal way of learning about this method of treatment. However, this is an ideal that may be difficult to achieve. Psychology departments and speech and language therapy departments are not always a short flight of stairs apart and the speech and language therapist may not always have access to an interested and willing psychologist. If speech and language therapists specialising in voice are to gain competence in using psychological methods in their work, they may have to find other opportunities or seek other ways of being exposed to a similar sort of learning experience. Experiential workshops, training days, and short courses can be a start but voice therapists will still have to find some way of obtaining psychological supervision with on-going cases. At this stage there are no easy and quick solutions to these challenges. However, as our understanding of psychogenic voice disorder expands, the authors are hopeful that ways will be found to train and support voice therapists in the use of psychological techniques. In this context, the authors' offer this volume as a small contribution to the training of therapists and hope it will provide new ideas and practical material for therapists working with individuals who cannot find the means within themselves to voice what they feel.

PETER BUTCHER
ANNIE ELIAS
LESLEY CAVALLI
London and Canterbury, 8 December, 2006

ACKNOWLEDGEMENTS

We would like to pay tribute to the very many patients who have shared so much of themselves and who have been our inspiration.
Additionally we would like to dedicate this book to our families:

To Bernice, Luke and Adam for their always stimulating love and companionship.

Peter

To Paul, who is my rock, for his unwavering support. To my children, Lucy, Clemmie and Izzy for their tolerance and their humour.

Annie

To my husband Philip, for his belief in me and constant support, and to my precious boys, Miles and Rory who were only dreams at the start of this project but have since 'sat' tolerantly, as honorary members, through many book meetings. Thanks also to other family members, friends and professional colleagues who have continued to inspire, encourage and advise me along the journey so far.

Lesley

1 Psychogenic Voice Disorders – A New Model

Speech and language therapists face challenges both in recognising when their patient has a psychogenic voice disorder and in knowing how to manage the case effectively. To get to this point it is necessary to understand what is meant by psychogenic voice disorder, to be informed about common aetiological features of this group of patients and to know how to make a competent assessment. At this stage it is necessary to have a clear idea, from evidence-based practice, as to how this population might respond to therapy and what treatment strategies are likely to be of value.

Despite agreeing that this small group of patients exists, the literature has to date been confusing about both terminology and classification and there are a limited number of reports of evidence-based treatment protocols. There is nervousness amongst speech and language therapists around both confident diagnosis and subsequent management.

In this chapter we set out a working model of psychogenic voice disorders (PVDs) as a guide to the clinician working in this area. We provide the speech and language therapist (SLT) with a framework for recognising and classifying this patient group. In subsequent chapters we will offer guidance to the speech and language therapist in assessing and managing these voice disorders within a psychological framework that incorporates clinical supervision. We also provide an explanation for when, in some complex cases, psychological referral is indicated.

A DEFINITION OF PSYCHOGENIC VOICE DISORDER

Drawing from previous definitions and classification systems, it is our view that a **psychogenic voice disorder** is a dysphonia (impaired or disordered voice) or aphonia (absent voice) where the causative or perpetuating factors are largely of psychological or emotional conflict. The voice problem may manifest itself with musculoskeletal tension and hyperkinetic behaviours and these may eventually give rise to laryngeal pathology, these being products or symptoms of the underlying psychological cause and the process of conversion.

What is critical here is that a confident diagnosis is reached only through careful psychological evaluation. A diagnosis of psychogenic voice disorder must not be made simply by *exclusion* of laryngeal pathology, in the way that the terms functional or non-organic might be employed. It is, of course, essential to have clarified the nature of any organic pathology through detailed laryngoscopic and preferably stroboscopic examination, however, the presence of negative results does not by default imply psychogenic causes. Assessment must be *inclusive* of psychological factors to a critical level and have clarified the causative and perpetuating role of these factors before diagnosis can be confirmed. The psychological evaluation will be outlined in Chapter 4.

Since musculoskeletal tension is a feature common to these voice disorders, we have said before that, 'the decision as to whether a voice disorder might be termed hyperkinetic or hyperfunctional rather than psychogenic is more a question of the degree to which underlying emotional stresses contribute to the dysphonia and of the degree of influence that those stresses have in perpetuating patterns of excessive laryngeal tension' (Butcher et al. 1993, p. 4).

PHYSIOLOGICAL AND PERCEPTUAL FEATURES
OF PSYCHOGENIC VOICE DISORDERS

Although there is overlap in the presenting phonatory and laryngeal signs and symptoms between muscle tension dysphonias and psychogenic dysphonias, there are often some features that are specific to a psychogenic dysphonia and are therefore helpful to the diagnosis. The phonatory and laryngeal signs and symptoms of a psychogenic aphonia are more diagnostically conclusive, and there are few types of voice disorder that present so dramatically.

Tables 1.1 and 1.2 illustrate the common presentations of psychogenic voice disorders and further helpful description can be found in Mathieson's text (2001, pp. 197–201).

Table 1.1: Physiological and perceptual features of psychogenic dysphonia

---

Phonatory Signs and Symptoms

- Perceptual features *may be* similar to muscle tension dysphonia.
- It may be inconsistent with clinical examination i.e. significantly abnormal voice despite absence of laryngeal pathology or only mild pathology.
- Variable voice, which may be normal during laughing/crying yet abnormal in conversation, and may be worse according to emotional context of speech.
- Dysphonia may be episodic.
- SLT may facilitate immediate normal voice.

Physiological Presentation, may be various, for example:

- 'normal' larynx i.e. no laryngeal pathology or neuropathology
- normal laryngeal function on a cough, laugh, breath hold
- incomplete vocal fold adduction or a glottic chink
- bowing of vocal folds
- hyperadduction of vocal folds
- supraglottic constriction i.e. ventricular band involvement and anterior-posterior squeezing
- laryngeal pathology (e.g. nodules)

Vocal Profile
May be forced, breathy, weak, with harshness or creak. May be in falsetto and may have pitch and phonation breaks. May have variable dysphonia interspersed with normal voice.

Table 1.2: Physiological and perceptual features of psychogenic aphonia

---

Phonatory Signs and Symptoms

- loss of voice of sudden onset
- may have had frequent and increasing aphonic episodes; may have had immediate aphonia
- may have occasional squeaks of voice
- usually normal vegetative behaviours
- SLT may facilitate immediate normal voice

Physiological Presentation, may be various, for example:

- incomplete vocal fold adduction
- glottic chink
- hyperadducted ventricular band
- bowing of vocal folds
- normal adduction for cough

Vocal Profile

- whisper
- sometimes only mouthing
- usually a normal cough, grunt etc.

COMMON AETIOLOGICAL FACTORS OF PSYCHOGENIC VOICE DISORDERS

Before presenting our model let us remind ourselves of other contributing evidence that has shaped our thinking. We can now draw on much research and literature that informs us about the aetiological features of these voice disorders. Psychogenic voice disorders are frequently multifactorial and have common factors, which we have summarised in Table 1.3. We will elaborate on these features when discussing assessment in Chapter 4. Appreciating the psychological aetiology of these voice disorders and being able to positively identify the aetiological features is critical in leading the speech and language therapist to a confident diagnosis and treatment of psychogenic voice disorder. Thus, a psychogenic voice disorder is confirmed provided that, first, a primary organic process has been carefully eliminated and second, that psychological aetiological features are identified alongside the phonatory and laryngeal presentations described above.

This assessment of the aetiological features is essential for the SLT because a diagnosis of psychogenic voice disorder implies that 'for true resolution, predisposing, precipitating and perpetuating psycho-emotional or psychosocial issues will need to be explored and addressed' (Baker 2002, pp. 84–5).

LOW MOOD/DEPRESSION AS AN AETIOLOGICAL FEATURE

In addition to the features described in Table 1.3 we have found that patients with psychogenic voice disorders frequently present with lowered mood or mild–moderate

Table 1.3: Common aetiological features of psychogenic voice disorders

Stressful life events and anxiety	Usually either follow an event of acute stress or are associated with stressful events over a long period of time. Anxiety and physical tension is an extremely common symptom. (Butcher et al. 1987; House and Andrews 1988; Kinzl et al. 1988; Freidl et al. 1990; Aronson 1990a; Gerritsma 1991; Roy et al. 1997; Deary et al. 1997; Andersson and Schalen 1998; Baker 1998; Mathieson 2001)
Common to females	More predominantly a female condition; approximately 8:1 females to male. (Aronson et al. 1966; Brodnitz 1969; House and Andrews 1987; Greene and Mathieson 1989; Gerritsma 1991; White et al. 1997; Millar et al. 1999)
Family and interpersonal difficulties	Frequently embroiled in family and interpersonal conflicts and experience difficulties with communication in these relationships. (Butcher et al. 1987; Andersson and Schalen 1998)
Difficulty expressing views and emotions	Person has considerable difficulties with assertiveness and the expression of inner feelings in specific situations. 'Conflict over speaking out' is a common feature. (Butcher et al. 1987; House and Andrews 1988; Kinzl et al. 1988; Freidl et al. 1990; Gerritsma 1991; Austin 1997; Andersson and Schalen 1998)
Suppressing anger and frustration	Being unable to express anger and frustration is the main inner conflict. Person is usually aware of a conflict but is coping by suppressing emotions and therefore not verbalising the anger. (Aronson et al. 1966; Butcher et al. 1987; House and Andrews 1988; Aronson 1990a)
Burden of responsibility	Taking on or trying to cope with above-average personal responsibilities. (Butcher et al. 1987)
Over-commitment and helplessness	Along with a tendency to be over-committed with responsibilities and in their family and social networks, they feel powerless about making personal change or changing the current situation. (Butcher et al. 1987; House and Andrews 1988; Andersson and Schalen 1998)
Near normal psychological adjustment	Not usually individuals who have a serious psychological disturbance. Not more than about 5% with a 'hysterical conversion' disorder. However, may be vulnerable to anxiety symptoms and have a tendency to somatise. (Aronson et al. 1966; House and Andrews 1987; Butcher et al. 1987; Aronson 1990; Gerritsma 1991; White et al. 1997; Millar et al. 1999)

depression. Common signs and symptoms are tearfulness, reported low mood, preoccupation with negative thoughts and feelings of helplessness and hopelessness.

Many authors note depression accompanying psychogenic voice disorders, for example pioneering studies by Guze and Brown (1962) and Aronson et al. (1966) showed their population to have a high degree of neurotic anxiety or depression. House and Andrews (1987) found only a small percentage, 16%, of their dysphonic population to be depressed, whereas a smaller study by Kinzl et al. (1988) found almost 50% to have a depressive neurasthenic syndrome. More recently Deary et al. (1997) found dysphonic women to have more anxiety and depression than either healthy or general practice controls. In 1999 Millar et al. found dysphonic women scored higher than controls on the depression subscales of the HADS (Hospital Anxiety and Depression Scale). Mathieson (2001) also describes depression associated with psychogenic disorder.

We have not included low mood or depression as a direct aetiological feature of psychogenic voice disorders because it can not be clearly determined whether the depression contributed to the voice disorder or whether it followed. In many cases we would suggest that the low mood or depression is secondary to the voice disorder. The person feels low because inner conflicts have not been resolved, and because the voice disorder frequently has a handicapping effect by preventing the person from performing normally, often having a negative impact on work and reducing social integration. In many circumstances they are grieving over the loss of normal voice function and are experiencing feelings of helplessness – features commonly associated with depression. However, given that many have been experiencing interpersonal difficulties and have difficulty expressing feelings, it would not be surprising if their lowered mood emerged in this context and became evident prior to voice loss. If this is the case, voice loss then becomes yet another thing to be depressed about.

Severe clinical depression is rarely seen in this population and we discuss this separately in Chapter 9.

UPPER RESPIRATORY TRACT INFECTION AS AN
AETIOLOGICAL FEATURE

Despite the fact that psychogenic voice disorders are typically characterised by normal laryngoscopic findings, clinicians will be familiar with case histories that relate colds and upper respiratory tract infections to the time of onset of the voice disorder.

There is a view expressed by some authors, for example Kinzl et al. (1988), that where a psychodynamic conflict already exists it is likely to be somatised at the site of least physical resistance. If a patient becomes overtaxed by a chronic stress situation, physical symptoms may develop at a site already weakened by infection. Furthermore, these authors also note that infections often occur or become worse during stress situations and that psychological factors have an influence on immunocompetence.

Other authors, for example Andersson and Schalen (1998), believe that the upper respiratory tract infection (URTI) only acts as a precipitating factor to the voice disorder, by provoking defensive laryngeal mechanisms. However, it seems that all authors are agreed that there is no direct causal link between the upper respiratory tract infection and the psychogenic voice disorder.

A NEW CLASSIFICATION SYSTEM FOR PSYCHOGENIC VOICE DISORDERS

We now present our model of classification for psychogenic voice disorders, summarised in Table 1.4. What now follows is the theoretical framework that underpins this model.

While our classification for psychogenic voice disorders has drawn on Freud's concept of conversion (the view that a psychological conflict is converted into a physical symptom), it has been reformulated to take into account the common aetiological features found in this population. The research supporting these findings and our own clinical impressions is the result of our work as clinical psychologist and speech and language therapists for over 20 years. Our classification has some common ground with previous classification systems, and, for example, it is sympathetic to Aronson's view (1990a) that these patients manifest psychologic disequilibrium, that the laryngeal muscles hypercontract in response to emotional stress and that the personality or emotional factors are the driving force of the problem. Our view that diagnosis depends upon an assessment that is inclusive of positive psychological factors to a critical level is also the position taken by Morrison and Rammage (1993) in their classification. Aronson expresses a similar position: 'A psychogenic voice disorder is broadly synonymous with a functional one but has the advantage of stating positively, based on an exploration of its causes, that the voice disorder is a manifestation of one or more types of psychologic disequilibrium, such as anxiety, depression, conversion reaction or personality disorder, that interfere with normal volitional control over phonation' (1990a, p. 121).

HYSTERICAL CONVERSION

Applying Freud's hysterical conversion label to psychogenic voice disorders is not straightforward. First of all, while his concept of conversion is valuable and should be retained, we take the view that Freud placed too much emphasis on the way the conversion resulted from unconscious sexual or aggressive conflicts, the way these conflicts are controlled by repression, and the way the conversion or behavioural response is reinforced socially by secondary gains. Second, taken as a whole, studies in the field of voice tell us that at maximum less than half the psychogenic population have

Table 1.4: The model

• Type 1: Classical Hysterical Conversion
• Type 2: Cognitive-Behavioural Conversion
• Type 3: Psychogenic-Habituated

features that fit Freud's diagnostic criteria for hysterical conversion and it may be as few as 4–5% (Aronson et al. 1966; Butcher et al. 1987; House and Andrews 1987; Gerritsma 1991). This evidence makes the term hysterical conversion an inappropriate classification for all psychogenic voice disorders. Thus, although the use of the rather outdated term **hysterical conversion** – or as we prefer **classical conversion** – does seem to have a place in the context of voice, the term is not interchangeable with psychogenic as a classification and appears useful for only a minority of patients. If used specifically the term hysterical conversion should be reserved for use when the psychological processes or diagnostic criteria of a traditional Freudian conversion disorder are present. This diagnostic difficulty has led us to propose a new application of the term conversion in the context of psychogenic voice disorders.

INTRODUCING TWO TYPES OF CONVERSION VOICE DISORDERS

The classification that we put forward is for clinicians to look more closely at the psychological processes that have contributed to the patient's voice disorder and to consider two distinct types of conversion (Butcher 1995).

Our opinion is that conversion disorders need not imply the full-blown Freudian hysterical conversion psychological processes. This model is supported by the current psychiatric criteria for conversion disorder in the Diagnostic and Statistics Manual (DSM-IV-TR), (American Psychiatric Association 2000). The DSM-IV criteria requires the initiation or exacerbation of the symptom to be preceded by psychological conflicts or other stressors. However, the DSM criteria no longer require the symptoms to represent a symbolic resolution of an unconscious psychological conflict, reducing anxiety and serving to keep the conflict out of awareness ('primary gain'). Neither do the criteria require the individual to derive benefit or secondary gain, and the feature of *la belle indifference* is not an essential requirement. Thus, modern thinking is that the term **conversion disorder** is used to represent a wide category and that a hysterical conversion is considered as one manifestation or sub-category of conversion disorder. Furthermore, in terms of Freud's initial model of conversion disorder having its origin in the repression of unacceptable sexual or aggressive impulses, it should be mentioned that these days most contemporary psychoanalysts would also acknowledge that the repression of *any* unacceptable anxiety feeling or thought can lead to a conversion disorder. This is reflected in the current DSM's wider interpretation of conversion.

Conversion Disorder – DSM-IV-TR Definition

The current diagnostic criteria for conversion disorder (DSM-IV) includes the following factors:

- The essential feature is the presence of symptoms or deficits affecting voluntary motor or sensory function that suggest a neurological or other general medical condition.
- Conflicts or other stressors precede the symptom or deficit.

- The symptom or deficit is not intentionally produced or feigned and, after appropriate investigation, it cannot be fully explained by a general medical condition.
- Furthermore, the symptom or deficit causes clinically significant distress or impairment in social, occupational or other important areas of functioning.

Thus, we can draw on the studies of psychogenic voice disorders and the current psychiatric diagnostic criteria, both outlined above, to distinguish between two types of conversion. The distinction of the two types of conversion is introduced below.

TYPE 1: CLASSICAL HYSTERICAL CONVERSION

- It fulfils the DSM criteria for a conversion of psychological stress into a physical symptom.
- Symptoms like *la belle indifference* or difficulty in consciously accessing unacceptable feelings suggest the *repression* of emotional conflicts.
- The primary gain is that repression removes the unpleasant conflict or feelings from consciousness.
- Some secondary gain from others, such as increased attention and concern, is likely to exist and acts as another powerful reinforcer of the conversion reaction.

TYPE 2: COGNITIVE BEHAVIOURAL CONVERSION

- It fulfils the DSM criteria for a conversion of psychological stress into a physical symptom.
- Conversion of psychological stress into a physical symptom is the apparent result of trying to *suppress* anxiety associated with emotional conflicts.
- The primary gain is avoidance of the feared consequences of acting on feelings.
- There are likely to be few compensatory secondary gains.

The two types of patients in this model experience a conversion of a psychological conflict into a physical symptom, but the nature of the inner conflict is different in each type and furthermore the person's coping mechanism will be different for each type, as we shall see in Table 1.5.

The model can be applied equally well to aphonics and to dysphonics. The determining factor as to which type a patient falls within, depends on a careful assessment that fully appreciates the psychological history and the presenting signs and symptoms. As described above, we have labelled these two groups of conversion voice disorders as Type 1 and Type 2. Type 1 represents what appears to be the minority of patients who fit a traditional Freudian hysterical conversion classification. The remainder and larger group of patients, 95%, fall into Type 2, who also experience a conversion of anxiety into physical symptoms, i.e. the voice disorder, but this conversion process is of a different order than that described by Freud. The distinction of the psychological processes at work in each group is described more fully in Table 1.5.

Table 1.5: Psychogenic conversion voice disorders – distinguishing features of the two main types

Type 1 Classical hysterical conversion (Traditional Freudian model. Rare, approx 5%)	Type 2 Cognitive behavioural conversion (Psychosocial/cognitive-behavioural model. Common, approx 95%)
1. Individual predisposed to problems by personality type, life experiences, traumas, social taboos around *expressing aggression/sexuality* and does not cope well with the presence of unacceptable or threatening emotions.	1. Individual predisposed to problems by personality type, life experiences, traumas, social taboos around *assertiveness* and the *expression of feelings,* which lead to lowered self-expression, self-esteem and feelings of powerlessness.
2. Exposure to negative life events or conflicts surrounding verbal expression of sexuality or aggression.	2. Exposure to negative life events or conflicts surrounding verbal expression of feelings.
3. Personality: uses *repression* and denial as coping mechanisms.	3. Personality: uses *suppression* or more conscious inhibition as a coping mechanism.
4. Repression eliminates awareness of the conflict and awareness of anxiety. This makes treatment more difficult because the cause is not accessible to the patient and therapist.	4. Suppression does not resolve conflicts, so the person continues to experience conflicts and the anxiety they cause. However, because they are near the surface the conflicts are easily accessible to patient and therapist.
5. The unconscious conflict is converted into physical symptoms, which outwardly symbolise the nature of the conflict.	5. The anxiety and inhibition becomes channelled or converted into musculoskeletal tension, much of which is focused on the site or battleground of the conflict, i.e. verbal expression.
6. The condition provides primary gains (avoidance of inner conflict, the experience of anxiety and the consequences of acting on the sexual or aggressive impulse) as well as secondary gains or reinforcements, which help maintain the condition.	6. Some primary gains (the person avoids the feared consequences of expressing feelings, but they cannot fully avoid the anxiety except to gain some relief through actively or consciously suppressing the conflict). The conversion of the conflict into a physical disorder causes additional anxieties and any secondary gains rarely provide significant compensation.
7. Low motivation to change because the primary and secondary gains provide sufficient reinforcement to maintain the status quo.	7. High motivation to change because suppression, inhibition and conversion have not resolved either the conflict or the anxiety or provide significant secondary gains.

DEFINING THE MODEL

TYPE 1 CONVERSION (CLASSICAL HYSTERICAL CONVERSION)

With regard to psychogenic voice disorder, our view is that the traditional interpretation of conversion disorder may be valid in cases where there is evidence of more severe psychopathology in a combination of persistent or protracted aphonia, the patient's passive acceptance of the condition, poor compliance with treatment, bland denial of distress or *la belle indifférence*, and indications that the condition provides important primary and secondary gains. This we classify above as Type 1. Although this rarer type presents usually as aphonia, we have seen this occasionally in patients with psychogenic dysphonia, typically with a tense, strained, falsetto voice. Other voice clinicians describe this Type 1 category. Mathieson (2001, pp. 199 and 205) acknowledges that only a small number of aphonics develop a true conversion symptom aphonia and fewer still will present with a true conversion symptom dysphonia. When Aronson describes conversion voice disorders (Aronson, 1990a, pp. 129–134), resulting in both aphonia and dysphonia, he too refers to the classical Freudian conversion disorder. In their classification system Morrison and Rammage (1993) describe briefly conversion aphonia and dysphonia that would probably fit the true Type 1 category.

Importantly, a Type 1 (classical Freudian hysterical conversion disorder) is extremely resistant to therapy because, unfortunately, the combination of repression and denial with primary and secondary gains makes the condition difficult to treat. Psychoanalysis was developed specifically as a treatment which would – through free association, the therapeutic transference and deepening insight – help the patient resolve the unconscious conflict at the heart of their problem, yet even analysts acknowledge that this population has a poor prognosis. It is fortunate that this is a rare complaint.

Joan a 53-year-old married mother of three grown up children presented with a 4-year history of dysphonia and episodic aphonia. ENT investigations had revealed a normal larynx with no pathology. The onset of this voice disorder followed shortly after an urgently arranged operation to remove a lump on her tongue. Despite the real possibility of the lump being cancer, she could not recall being afraid or concerned for her wellbeing at this time.

Similarly, despite having moderately high scores for anxiety and depression as determined on the Hospital Anxiety and Depression Scale, Joan also denied any current awareness of anxiety or emotional stress. Furthermore, despite some evidence to the contrary, she denied experiencing any conflicts over speaking out or difficulties in expressing her feelings or experiencing any burden of responsibility. Thus, the psychological assessment confirmed Joan's use of **repression** or **denial** as a mechanism of defence for coping with emotional conflicts and anxiety typical of a Type 1 (classical hysterical) conversion. This tendency to use repression and therefore her lack of insight into her thoughts and feelings made it difficult to offer Joan treatment.

For full case details see Chapter 10, pages 178–80.

A case study by Baker (1998) illustrates the complexities of treating a true Type 1 conversion dysphonia.

TYPE 2 COGNITIVE BEHAVIOURAL CONVERSION

By contrast, the majority of patients with psychogenic voice loss appear to be suffering from symptoms of musculoskeletal tension and anxiety caused by life stress and interpersonal conflicts that frequently involve difficulty expressing feelings. Although their distress is converted into a physical loss or impairment of voice, and while inhibited or suppressed anger may play an important role, these patients fit more comfortably within the modern classification of conversion disorder rather than the classical Freudian interpretation. Aronson (1990a) describes these psychogenic voice disorders within a broad category of musculoskeletal tension voice disorders and Mathieson (2001) classifies them as stress-related dysphonia or aphonia. We propose calling this group a Type 2 cognitive behavioural conversion voice disorder; they form the great majority of the psychogenic voice disorders found in speech and language therapists' caseloads. We have chosen to label this type as 'cognitive behavioural' since popular use of the term 'psychosomatic' has negative associations and other more descriptive terms such as 'psycho-social-biological' are too unwieldy. The label cognitive behavioural does imply the interplay between psychological process and the physical/behavioural responses, although it may not adequately highlight the social and biological features. The Type 2 patient may include both the psychogenic dysphonic and aphonic and probably explains why the majority of aphonics do return to normal voice relatively quickly with an experienced voice therapist. Mathieson describes this type of psychogenic aphonic (2001, pp. 199–200) as being tense, anxious and distressed by their aphonia, near to tears, overburdened, and with a history of stressful life events. Both Aronson (1990a) and Mathieson (2001) report a good prognosis for patients who can develop insight into the psychosomatic basis of the aphonia. These views closely reflect our own experience with this population.

Although some authors take the view (Aronson et al. 1966) that the secondary gain of the voice disorder provides attention from others in the majority of patients and while Freud's model emphasises that secondary gain is a feature of Type 1, we have found the secondary gain is usually quite negligible or non-existent for Type 2.

In contrast to the poor prognosis afforded to the Type 1 classical Freudian conversion patient, there are grounds to be optimistic about treating the more common forms of conversion disorder causing aphonia or dysphonia. Psychodynamic treatment might benefit this group (Type 2) by helping the individual understand the suppressed emotional impact of early traumas that have predisposed them to inner conflicts, causing such things as low self-esteem, feelings of powerlessness and difficulties with assertiveness. Alternatively, therapists treating this group might employ cognitive behaviour therapy (CBT). This approach would commonly emphasise the role of unconscious schemas (core constructs about the self, world and other people), the way dysfunctional cognitions (rules for living, underlying assumptions, automatic thoughts) shape emotions and behaviour, and would focus on practical strategies like stress management and role-playing techniques to help the person control anxiety, improve communication skills and be more assertive.

The case of Sue, a 42-year-old, who presented with a falsetto dysphonia of sudden onset, illustrates a Type 2 (psychogenic cognitive behavioural) dysphonia that resolved quickly through a combination of CBT assessment/treatment techniques and symptomatic voice therapy.

Initially Sue attributed her voice loss to laryngitis, although she did not identify any URTI. However, through a careful psychosocial interview she identified significant emotional stresses and conflicts throughout the preceding year and immediately preceding the dysphonia. Sue had experienced a traumatic year during which her husband had an affair and left her. She had experienced high anxiety levels and had attempted suicide. She explained that her husband continued to dominate her and regularly let himself into the house. She wanted to move on but she was financially bound to him and she felt powerless with him. Sue felt angry towards her husband, because of his betrayal, his dominance and because of the prospect of losing her home. In the weeks preceding her dysphonia she had become increasingly unhappy at work and in particular with her boss. She knew that he too was having an affair and that she had transferred a lot of the anger she felt towards her husband onto her boss, causing difficulties in the work place.

Understanding the link between emotional stress and voice loss enabled Sue to quickly understand the causal features of her dysphonia and to develop self-insight. This insight allowed Sue to move forward, to set herself targets to behave more assertively with her husband and to make positive plans for her future. Symptomatic voice therapy helped to re-establish modal voice; however, the quick resolution was attributed primarily to Sue's insight and understanding and her ability to think and behave differently as a consequence.

For full case details see Chapter 10, pages 191–4.

Considering psychogenic aphonia within this model of Type 1 and Type 2 may help throw more light on observations recorded in earlier voice studies. For example, in 1969 Brodnitz described a large study of 74 aphonics. Of the 53 patients who entered therapy, all but 2 recovered normal voices, 44 doing so during the first therapy session; the remainder requiring an average of 4–6 sessions to restore normal voice. Seventeen of the patients went on to receive psychotherapy to help with severe emotional conflicts. One case was resolved finally through hypnosis and only one case was intractable despite voice therapy and psychotherapy. We would postulate that a closer examination of the psychological profile of these 53 patients might reveal a majority who would fulfil our Type 2 criteria with a minority, perhaps only the two, fulfilling the classical Freudian Type 1.

The distinction between Type 1 and Type 2 certainly helps to explain why in the majority of cases a confident speech and language therapist will be able to guide an aphonic to a quick return to normal voice, frequently within the initial session, while there is a minority of cases where this is not possible and despite exhausting the clinician's repertoire of behavioural tricks and counselling skills the aphonia remains intractable. Although some of these more complex aphonics will fall within a Type 2 conversion and will probably resolve with the help of skilled psychological support, it is within this hard-to-treat group that there will be a rarer Type 1 conversion disorder. We will offer an approach to managing the return of voice for Type 2 aphonic in Chapter 5 (pages 90–7).

With our knowledge of the aetiological features of psychogenic voice disorders described earlier, we can now individually attribute these to the Type 1 or the Type 2 conversion group. The distinguishing aetiological features of each group are detailed in Table 1.6.

DISTINGUISHING FEATURES OF TYPE 1 AND TYPE 2

To summarise from our classification system there are key distinguishing features between Type 1 and Type 2.

PREDISPOSITION TO PSYCHOLOGICAL PROBLEMS/PERSONALITY TYPE

Both types of patient may have life experiences and traumas that make them vulnerable to problems. In particular Type 1 is likely to have experienced family or social taboos around the expression of aggression, sexuality or other unacceptable or taboo emotions while Type 2 will probably have encountered taboos around the expression of assertiveness, feelings or views. However, what really distinguishes the two groups is their personality and coping strategies. The Type 1 personality uses *repression* as a mechanism of defence and, eventually, turns a blind eye to stress. Type 2 on the other hand reacts emotionally to stress, tries unsuccessfully to *suppress* emotions and, as a result, tends to establish anxiety driven patterns of behaviour.

The Trigger/conflict

In a typical case, according to Freud, the trigger for the Type 1 conversion will be around an exposure to a life event or conflict surrounding the verbal expression of sexuality or aggression. The conflict becomes the fear of acting on a sexual or aggressive urge. Because this is unconscious, we have no proof that this is going on

Table 1.6: Distinguishing aetiological features of conversion
Type 1 and Type 2 psychogenic voice disorders

Conversion Type 1 or 2	Aetiological Features	
1 and 2	Stress and anxiety	Usually either follows an event of acute stress or is associated with stress over a long period of time. Anxiety and physical tension is an extremely common symptom.
1 and 2	Common to females	It is predominantly a female condition.
1 and 2	Family and interpersonal difficulties	Frequently embroiled in family and interpersonal difficulties.
1 and 2	Difficulty expressing views and emotions	The person has considerable difficulties with assertiveness and the expression of inner feelings in specific situations.
1 = repressing 2 = suppressing	Repressing or suppressing uncomfortable emotions	Expressing anger and frustration or finding it difficult to handle unacceptable emotions is the main inner conflict. Type 1: Unaware of conflict because repression has made it unconscious. Type 2: Aware of conflict but coping by suppressing emotions.
2	Burden of responsibility	Taking on, or trying to cope with above average personal responsibilities.
2	Over-commitment and helplessness	A tendency to be over-committed with responsibilities and in their social networks and feeling powerless about making personal change or changing the current situation.
2	Near normal psychological adjustment	Not usually individuals who have a serious psychological disturbance.

but can only assume something very conflicting is occurring for the person to be caught up in the act of repression. It must be stressed here – as an extension of Freud's initial formulation – that modern day psychoanalysts believe that the conflict may involve unacceptable feelings other than sex and aggression. The case of Joan (see earlier case study, page 10 and Chapter 10, pages 178–80) is a good example. The evidence indicated that what she was repressing when the dysphonia began was not sexual or aggressive feelings. It was the unacceptable thought of very likely having cancer and possibly dying. Yalom (1980), for example, has made a strong case for viewing fear of death and meaninglessness as a cause of psychopathology (see also Butcher, 1984, for a further discussion with case examples of the way fear of death or preoccupation with mortality can be a cause of clinically significant anxiety and symptoms of depression).

Typically, the trigger for the Type 2 conversion seems to be exposure to a life event or events that increase feelings of powerlessness or conflicts around the verbal expression of feelings which may include anger. The conflict is the difficulty in expressing feelings or the conflict over speaking out experienced by the person.

Coping Mechanism

The coping mechanism for a person in Type 1 is an unconscious repression and denial of the conflict. The process of repression effectively eliminates the conflict and any awareness of anxiety, thus the person is satisfactorily free from distress and will often show little concern for their symptoms, or *la belle indifference*. Conversely, the coping mechanism for a person in Type 2 is a more conscious suppression of the conflict. Suppression does not resolve or fully remove the conflict from consciousness so the person continues to experience the conflicts and the anxiety that they cause:

The Conversion

In both Type 1 and Type 2 the conflict is converted into physical symptoms, the malfunctioning voice; in both groups the conversion itself does symbolise the type of conflict. In Type 1 the significance of the voice loss is that it prevents the person from either expressing sexually unacceptable feelings or speaking about other taboo subjects like death or meaninglessness or, more commonly, verbally expressing feelings of anger or outrage; it is therefore symbolic of these unconscious conflicts and governed by the operation of repression. In Type 1 and 2 the anxiety and inhibition resulting from the conflict is converted into musculoskeletal tension, mostly around the larynx. Thus the conversion is focused on the site or battleground of the conflict; however, in Type 2 it is usually symbolic of the difficulty in showing assertiveness or feelings of self-expression and is created by the action of suppression and the physical inhibition of voice.

Primary and Secondary Gains

The conversion for Type 1 provides both primary and secondary gains that are reinforcing. The primary gains include the avoidance of the inner conflict, anxiety and the consequences of acting on the sexual or aggressive impulse. Secondary gains exist as a consequence of the voice disorder, for example, avoiding responsibilities or gaining the solicitous and caring behaviour of others.

There are some partial primary gains for Type 2, namely the person avoids the feared consequences of expressing true feelings. However, because the conflict is only inhibited or suppressed, the person continues to experience the anxiety. Furthermore, the voice disorder itself tends to cause additional anxiety and any secondary gains rarely provide significant compensation.

AND TYPE 3

To complete the picture we need to discuss patients with a non-organic dysphonia who do not entirely fit the Type 1 or 2 groups and we believe are in fact a subgroup of Type 2. We have outlined the distinguishing features of all three types in Table 1.7.

Table 1.7: Comparing the distinguishing features of the three PVD types

Type 1 Classical (hysterical) Conversion	Type 2 Cognitive-behavioural Conversion	Type 3 Habituated Conversion
(Traditional Freudian model. Rare, approx 5%)	(Psychosocial/cognitive-behavioural model. Common, approx 95%)	(Originating in Type 2 processes, which have largely resolved)
1. Individual predisposed to problems by personality type, life experiences, traumas, and social taboos around expressing aggression/sexuality.	1. Individual predisposed to problems by personality type, life experiences, traumas, social taboos around *assertiveness* and the *expression of feelings,* which lead to lowered self-expression, self-esteem and feelings of powerlessness.	1. Individual predisposed to problems by personality type, life experiences, traumas, social taboos around *assertiveness* and the *expression of feelings,* which lead to lowered self-expression, self-esteem and feelings of powerlessness.
2. Exposure to negative life events or conflicts surrounding verbal expression of sexuality or aggression.	2. Exposure to negative life events or conflicts surrounding verbal expression of feelings.	2. Exposure to negative life events or conflicts surrounding verbal expression of feelings.
3. Personality: uses *repression* and denial as coping mechanisms.	3. Personality: uses *suppression* or more conscious inhibition as a coping mechanism.	3. Personality: uses *suppression* or more conscious inhibition as a coping mechanism.
4. Repression eliminates awareness of the conflict and awareness of anxiety. This makes treatment more difficult because the cause is not accessible to the patient and therapist.	4. Suppression does not resolve conflicts, so the person continues to experience conflicts and the anxiety they cause. However, because they are 'near the surface' the conflicts are easily accessible to patient and therapist.	4. Suppression had not resolved conflicts but circum-stances have changed. The conflicts have resolved or greatly diminished so that there is no longer any need for suppression. The original conflict has been minimised and may be forgotten.

5. The unconscious conflict is converted into physical symptoms, which outwardly symbolise the nature of the conflict.

5. The anxiety and inhibition becomes channelled or converted into musculoskeletal tension, much of which is focused on the site or battleground of the conflict i.e. verbal expression.

5. The anxiety and inhibition was originally channelled or converted into musculoskeletal tension (MST) much of which was focused on the site or battleground of the conflict. Despite resolution of the conflict and anxiety the muscu-loskeletal tension (MST) becomes conditioned. Thus, the voice disorder is maintained out of habit.

6. The condition provides primary gains (avoidance of inner conflict, the experience of anxiety and the consequences of acting on the sexual or aggressive impulse) as well as secondary gains or reinforcements, which help maintain the condition.

6. Some primary gains (the person avoids the feared consequences of expressing feelings, but they cannot fully avoid the anxiety except to gain some relief through actively or consciously suppressing the conflict). The conversion of the conflicts into a physical disorder causes additional anxieties. Any secondary gains rarely provide significant compensation.

6. There is no longer any primary gain because the conflict has resolved. Any secondary gain is negligible in main-taining the problem.

7. Low motivation to change because the primary and secondary gains provide sufficient reinforcement to maintain the status quo.

7. High motivation to change because suppression, inhibition and conversion have not resolved either the conflict or the anxiety or provide significant secondary gains.

7. Psychological distress no longer driving high levels of motivation to get better. Motivation levels likely to be similar to larger population of muscle tension dysphonia (MTD) patients, including varying levels of distress over their voice loss.

TYPE 3: PSYCHOGENIC-HABITUATED VOICE DISORDER

These are the patients who started out with a psychogenic voice disorder but along the way the precipitating stressors or conflicts diminish or resolve yet the dysphonia or aphonia continues because of habituated behavioural patterns of voice use. These patients were not described in our earlier work but we believe they make up a small proportion of the 95% of patients with identified Type 2, cognitive behavioural conversion. Several authors describe these patients. Mathieson (2001) explains:

> Depending on the duration of the problem when the patient attends for treatment, the voice reflects not only the current psychological status of the individual but also vocal habit. In some instances the precipitating stressful event or circumstances have passed and the patient is no longer unduly stressed or distressed, but the kinaesthetic model for normal phonation cannot be retrieved and so the problem persists.
>
> (p.198)

The description by Brodnitz (1969), illustrates why aphonics in this group can be so successfully remediated. 'In many instances, particularly if the aphonia has persisted for a long time, the psychologic conflict that produced the aphonia may have lost its validity. The patient is quite ready to resume normal communication but he needs expert help to accomplish this' (p. 1249). This is why a firm authoritative approach by the speech therapist, guiding the patient through a sequence of graded behavioural tasks works well, with no need to become involved in an in-depth psychological interview.

This group of patients were certainly psychogenic in origin and would share the hyperkinetic muscle misuse patterns shared by all patients with psychogenic voice disorder. Despite the fact that the stressors have resolved or significantly diminished, the patient continues to have a voice disorder because it has become habituated into a pattern of muscle misuse.

A patient with dysphonia in this category would be Wendy, a 22-year-old who had a long-standing conflict expressing views to her mother. The voice disorder had its origin in an emotional conflict and the attempt to cope with the distress through suppression of the conflict (a Type 2 aetiology), the resulting anxiety causing increased musculoskeletal tension particularly of the laryngeal mechanism. This hyperkinetic voice pattern became strongly patterned over time. In Wendy's case her relationship with her mother considerably improved and the conflict resolved, yet the dysphonia persisted because it had become habituated. This was a voice disorder with a psychogenic cause, the psychogenic factors resolved but the behavioural features persisted as a result of habituation.

Recognising the presence of a psychogenic-habituated voice disorder also highlights the way in which both Types 1 and 2 are vulnerable to developing a faulty laryngeal muscle set through the practice of regularly misusing the voice.

TAKING ACCOUNT OF MAJOR TRAUMA

Within the common aetiological features of PVD we have cited wide-ranging references linking the onset of the voice disorder to stressful life events. This precipitating feature may be due to events and stress of the recent past or be linked to stressful events that have endured for some time. We have shown in our definition of Type 1 and Type 2 conversion voice disorders that there is a psychological coping mechanism of either repression or suppression of the stressful conflict. We now need to consider a conversion reaction that has in its origins a variation both in the type of the original stressor and in the psychological coping mechanism.

There is a body of evidence amongst psychologists working with victims of major trauma, that some individuals use **dissociation** as a means of repressing the traumatic event and removing it from consciousness. In these cases the traumatic event caused psychological stress of such a profound nature that the individual becomes dissociated from the experience, in other words the patient cannot bring to mind details of what happened or may even have no conscious memory of the event. It is now widely accepted for example, that dissociation in children who have suffered sexual abuse is common and may play a role in helping them cope with major traumatic events. Because the trauma is dissociated from consciousness there is also a dissociation from voluntary control that may result in a conversion reaction affecting motor or sensory systems.

It was Pierre Janet (1920) who first developed the concept of dissociation in connection with trauma. Initially Freud fully supported the view that terrifying traumatic events causing profound psychological distress – for which the person was unprepared – resulted in dissociation and led to a conversion reaction. Freud used this theoretical framework to explain the conversion disorders experienced by soldiers in the First World War when they experienced conversion aphonia or blindness. Freud later moved from this stand to develop his model of conversion related to unacceptable sexual and aggressive impulses, which we have reviewed in our description of Type 1 PVDs.

However, Janet's model continues to be of value currently in cognitive behavioural models of post-traumatic stress disorder (PTSD). He recognised that when some people were placed in an unbearable and frightening traumatic situation which evoked 'vehement emotions' that could not be integrated into personal understanding or awareness, the experience can become 'dissociated' or split off from consciousness. It was Janet's view that where the memory traces of the trauma have remained unexpressed they would become fixed and it is only through the traumatic experience being brought back fully into consciousness and told as a personal narrative that the traumatic experience can become integrated into the self, thus allowing the patient to process and come to terms with the experience. This explanatory model and treatment concept closely parallels contemporary views in cognitive behaviour therapy on the nature and treatment of PTSD; specifically, the emphasis on processing memories of the trauma through exposure, reliving and a focus on emotional 'hot spots' (see, for example, Ehlers & Clarke 2000; Grey et al. 2002).

In a recent publication Baker (2003) has presented thought-provoking evidence that in rare instances a psychogenic voice disorder can be linked to a forgotten traumatic event that may have occurred months or years prior to the onset of the voice disorder. In these cases Baker illustrates that a trigger reawakens the trauma and that this coincides with the onset of the voice disorder. Significantly the qualitative nature of the traumatic experience is represented in the somatisation of the voice disorder. The conversion or physical symptoms coalesce at the site of the trauma – in these cases, the throat, voice and airways. Baker uses Pierre Janet's model of dissociation and conversion to make sense of the psychological processes at work in these cases.

Using case studies, Baker describes the scenario of two patients with psychogenic voice disorder whose voice or full psychological recovery did not resolve through either symptomatic voice therapy or from attempts to recall recent stressful events or from a conflict over speaking out (as might be expected with a Type 2 patient). One of the patients presented with a psychogenic aphonia superimposed on a left vocal fold paresis. This required careful differential diagnosis and close liaison and consultation with the otolaryngologist. Through skilful therapeutic guidance both patients were able eventually to recall traumatic memories that had previously remained unconscious and unexpressed. These traumatic events varied in the time elapsed, from four months to 38 years. As part of the traumatic experience there was a direct threat to the throat, be it a fear of choking to death or an inability to cry out for help.

In each case a more recent stressful experience, which had some similarity or association with the earlier traumatic experience, reawakened memories and emotions of the original trauma and precipitated the voice loss. The validity of this is discussed by current experts in the treatment of PTSD (van der Kolk, McFarlane and Weisarth 1996) who explain that traumatised patients seem 'to react to reminders of the trauma with responses that had been relevant to the original threat' (p. 52). However, the dissociated state continues to prevent memory of the trauma from surfacing from the sub-conscious to consciousness.

These cases described by Baker do not fit comfortably with either a Type 1 classical Freudian conversion or Type 2 cognitive behavioural classification. For example, although apparently repressing the trauma they did not demonstrate features of *la belle indifference*; the repression was not related to fear of acting on a sexual or aggressive impulse, the conversion does not occur at the time of the initial trauma, and they were clearly motivated to resolve their voice problem.

What they do have in common with a Type 1 formulation, however, is that through the action of the unconscious process of repression and dissociation they have found a way of avoiding being conscious of an unacceptable experience and as a result, have been unable to either assimilate or accommodate the experience into their view of themselves, their world and the behaviour of others.

We have spent some time exploring this fascinating area because it may hold significant clues when patients with a psychogenic voice disorder do not make a full resolution, and where the patient does not fit with either the Type 1 Freudian conversion or with the Type 2 conversion and perhaps where the therapist suspects that 'the full story has not been told' (Baker 2003, p. 311). Assuming that the therapist has been vigilant in confirming, through liaison and review with ENT, that a primary organic diagnosis is not the cause, it may be important to consider in these minority of cases whether the origins of the voice disorder might lie in traumatic events experienced some time in the past and about which the patient has no conscious memory. Since the voice disorder in these cases seems to be triggered by an experience associated with the original trauma, the therapist should consider returning to detailed questioning about events around onset, encouraging patients to return in their mind's eye to the day their voice became problematic, and asking for as much detail as possible in the hope of touching on the trigger event or happening.

MUSCLE MISUSE VOICE DISORDER

This leaves the group of patients who clearly have developed a vocal abuse or misuse in the absence of significant psychological conflict or stress. This group will have its origin in the behavioural or functional use of the voice, such as in the case of professional voice users who are pushing their voice beyond healthy limits and without attention to good voice care.

We apply the term **muscle misuse voice disorder** within our classification system to refer solely to voice disorders that are associated with laryngeal muscle misuse and where there are no significant psychological factors in the origins of the voice disorder. Historically these might have been labelled 'functional' but we accept that this is an ambiguous label.

We would not deny that patients in this muscle misuse group may present with some degree of stress – perhaps having an inner pressure to perform well and be successful, perhaps having perfectionistic tendencies or the need to be in control coupled with performance anxiety or tension – but major psychological conflict and stress will not have been the primary aetiology or maintaining factor for this group. Of course, these patients will also experience their fair share of stressful life events; however, they will typically manage these stresses appropriately and not become overburdened by them, and they are likely to have good support networks from family or friends. In our experience it is true that these patients may demonstrate areas of over-commitment either in their work or in their social engagements, but this does not make a major contribution to negative emotional states. Our Type 2 conversion voice disorders, on the other hand, may present with very similar voices to this group and with similar hyperfunctional laryngeal patterns but they will have a positive psychological aetiology of more significant inner and interpersonal conflict. We acknowledge, however, that this is not always an easy distinction to make. It is often one of degree and it requires a sensitive psychosocial interview to arrive at a positive diagnosis.

The treatment for this group of patients will focus on behavioural voice therapy to unpick the faulty patterns of behaviour and re-establish good voice habits. There will be minimal attention to cognitive strategies required for this group.

Case studies demonstrating differences between a muscle misuse dysphonia and a Type 2 psychogenic cognitive behavioural dysphonia.

MUSCLE MISUSE DYSPHONIA

Jim was a 21-year-old presenting with swollen and oedematous vocal folds. He was determined to make a life as a singer and had begun to experience vocal strain when singing four months earlier when he had felt under the weather. Subsequently, he had noticed difficulties singing freely, a loss of his higher register and some hoarseness in his speaking voice. Jim presented with moderate harshness and increased laryngeal tension in his speaking voice, mildly raised loudness, a rapid rate of speech and a tendency to drive his voice on shallow breath support. He was extremely talkative and he was a heavy voice user. He sang in a rock/pop band as the only vocalist and also sang as a solo act. He was performing in up to four gigs a week in pub venues and was rehearsing twice a week. He described himself as a social animal and admitted to shouting with his mates. Jim had a slightly chaotic life style; he tended to stay up into the early hours of the morning, finding it hard to unwind after a gig. He was an occasional smoker of cigarettes and cannabis but drank little alcohol. Although Jim had quite recently parted from his long-term girlfriend, he was not distressed by this and viewed it as an opportunity to socialise more. He said that he found relaxation difficult and in the clinic he was a fidget. He threw himself enthusiastically into his voice therapy although his view was that a couple of sessions should fix his voice and he did not seem motivated for a full course of voice therapy.

The SLT classified Jim as having a muscle misuse dysphonia aggravated by some vocal abuse. Voice therapy was directed to two areas. First, to behavioural modifications around his voice use; namely reducing the number of gigs and rehearsals, pacing the gigs and changing the selection of some of the music, reducing his talking, eliminating shouting and slowing the rate of his speech. Second, to direct symptomatic voice therapy techniques, to establish centred breath, to free the body, to vocal deconstriction exercises and a free projected voice.

Jim attended three sessions of voice therapy. He made quick and successful modifications to his voice use and vocal behaviour in some areas but not in others, such as reducing his rate of speech. He reported improvements in his singing immediately; he no longer felt vocal strain or discomfort and was able to negotiate pitch changes in his music more easily. There continued to be features of harshness and slightly increased loudness in Jim's speaking voice but he felt further improvement was down to him practising. The therapist felt that a true resolution of the dysphonia was unlikely since Jim was not keen to commit to more voice therapy sessions. A laryngostroboscopic review in the voice clinic, three months after Jim's initial voice therapy assessment revealed a marked improvement with almost normal vocal folds.

TYPE 2 PSYCHOGENIC COGNITIVE BEHAVIOURAL

Cathy was a 42-year-old singer who was referred to speech and language therapy with increasing vocal strain during her singing performances, hoarseness after singing and oedematous vocal folds. She sang professionally in clubs, mostly rock and pop styles, typically one or two gigs each weekend as a solo vocalist. When assessed, Cathy was not dysphonic in her speaking voice but in voice exercises she demonstrated vocal strain with a marked increase in laryngeal tension, moderate breathiness and raised pitch. She had neck and shoulder tension and her larynx was tight to palpate.

Cathy smoked 25 cigarettes a day and had an alcohol dependency problem. She had a history of depression and had occasional suicidal thoughts. She had been in psychotherapy for a number of years (although recently she had not found this useful as it was not giving her solutions, and she said she was only going along so as not to let the trainee psychotherapist down). She had recognised that her singing was a mixed blessing; on the one hand it was an emotional release and she used the lyrics to express herself, on the other, if she felt the audience was not listening to her it would reinforce her feelings of poor self-worth and would trigger a depressive reaction. She said that for every good gig she would have one bad one. Cathy tended to jump to errors of thinking if her audience did not give warm appreciation. She would conclude that they did not like her or her voice and as well as feeling depressed she would then develop some performance anxiety and fear during the week before the next gig. Cathy also felt unhappy in her marriage but said that she didn't know how to resolve this. She tended to share few of her thoughts and emotions with her husband but would fall in with his view of things despite having her own opinions. She preferred not to 'rock the boat' but, as a consequence, she felt lonely in her marriage. This behaviour suggested the feature of 'conflict over speaking out'.

The SLT classified this patient as a Type 2 psychogenic voice disorder. She had run into problems of vocal misuse in her singing with obvious increased laryngeal tension and her use of alcohol and cigarettes were obviously unhealthy for her larynx. Significantly though, she was an emotionally vulnerable lady and her poor vocal technique in her singing was inextricably linked to her thoughts and emotions and in particular to whether she was liked by her audience.

A course of voice therapy was planned with three areas of focus. First, some symptomatic behavioural work directed towards freeing her body and vocal tract, establishing centred breath, experiencing some free voice and making practical changes to her music and to her voice care. Alongside this, cognitive behavioural therapy techniques were directed at challenging her negative assumptions about her audiences and changing these to positive self-statements, anxiety management and training in rapid relaxation and a more positive approach to her time management prior to a gig so that she could prepare herself both physically and emotionally. Finally, Cathy was encouraged to explore her behaviour of holding things back from her husband and to see that her tendency of falling in with his views would reinforce his belief that she was in agreement. Using some discussion of recent situations between them, the therapist was able to rehearse with Cathy ways that she could voice both her feelings and views and she began to reflect on the change that this would have on her husband's behaviour.

Cathy attended five sessions with the speech and language therapist. Progress was steady and sustained. She made sensible adjustments to her performances including changing the music and taking comfort breaks. She worked on her voice technique and incorporated a careful warm-up routine prior to singing. She practised changing her negative thinking about her audience to positive self-statements and became quite skilled in this technique. She began to enjoy her singing and look forward to her performances. She coped well with a less than generous audience and managed to use her positive thinking and was able to report afterwards that she sang well, despite the poor audience, and she did not feel low afterwards. By the time of her ENT review four months after her voice assessment, she was anticipating singing well and was finding her singing performance was much improved. She no longer had any anxiety about her voice and her vocal folds were normal on examination. Although she remained dissatisfied with her marriage, she recognised that she had a part to play in changing this. She opted to continue with psychotherapy which she said was becoming more useful.

THE TREATMENT OF CHOICE FOR PSYCHOGENIC VOICE DISORDERS

Although there have been few studies that investigate the long-term effects of therapy and the relapse rates for patients with psychogenic voice disorder, it has been reported that 5–10% do not show improvements with speech therapy (Brodnitz 1969; Koufman and Blalock 1982). In a survey of speech therapists in the UK in 1988 (Elias et al. 1989) a high proportion of therapists estimated the relapse rates of their psychogenic patients to be between 25 and 50%. The same survey found no standard psychological techniques in use and identified that 70% of therapists would welcome more training in the treatment of voice disorders from a clinical psychologist or psychiatrist. There was a clear trend in this survey for those therapists with a longer experience of treating psychogenic voice disorders to estimate that more sessions would be needed. These same voice specialists were undertaking significantly more work with psychologists and psychiatrists than non-specialist therapists. A more recent study (Andersson and Schalen 1998) provides some evidence that combining voice therapy with psychological methods gives good long-term resolution in both effectively treating the voice disorder and the emotional stress. Andersson and Schalen point out that cognitive behaviour therapy alone is not usually effective for psychogenic voice disorders, but when combined with voice therapy, results are good in the majority of cases. There have been many papers and studies advocating that speech therapists either work with or be trained by psychologists in the treatment of psychogenic voice disorders, for example: Hayward and Simmons 1982; Butcher and Elias 1983; Butcher et al. 1987; Aronson 1990b; Freeman 1991; Scott et al. 1997; Baker 1998. We are reminded by Baker's (2003) review of the literature that 'therapeutic approaches that seek to integrate re-instatement of the voice with an understanding of the sensitive relationship between the stressful events, relationship difficulties, and patterns of reticence in expressing negative emotions, generally lead to successful resolution of the psychogenic dysphonia' (p. 311).

In their review of the management of patients with functional dysphonia, Scott et al. (1997) advocate that clinical psychologists develop a training and consultative role for speech therapists, equipping them with additional psychological skills, leading to more effective treatment. They suggest that psychologists can make an important contribution as members of the voice clinic team. Although appreciating that psychologists can conduct psychological interviews, advise on treatment and perhaps offer cognitive behaviour therapy to this patient group, these authors suggest that they may have a greater role in training the speech and language therapists to treat these patients and to recognise when referral to mental health services is required. We would support this viewpoint.

THE TREATMENT OF CHOICE FOR TYPE 1 (CLASSICAL HYSTERICAL CONVERSION)

As we have said earlier, a Type 1 is unlikely to resolve. The speech and language therapist needs to be able to recognise these patients and to consult a psychiatrist or a clinical psychologist in order to plan an appropriate way of managing their care.

Identifying The Type 1 Conversion

There are features of the Type 1 personality and features of the conversion that may be quite transparent in the therapist's contact with the patient. These features provide helpful diagnostic signs for the speech and language therapist to be alert to a Type 1 patient. Typically this patient will be resistant to exploring a psychological cause for the voice disorder or to discussing emotional topics. The patient tends to 'want a fix' to the problem. Because of this low motivation for change (motivation would require an acknowledgement of the conflict) the patient does not take ownership of the voice problem and will put the responsibility for improving the voice onto the therapist. Consequently the patient may present as demanding and controlling. The patient's controlling behaviour is indicative of personality type and the repression of the inner conflict as a mechanism of defence. The patient may appear angry and frustrated but typically will not complain of anxiety and depression so commonly seen in the Type 2 cases. In some cases, despite being aphonic or having a significant dysphonia, patients can show a surprising lack of concern for the symptoms, i.e. *la belle indifference.*

In turn the therapist may find little empathy for this patient who seems to be someone with whom it is quite difficult to relate and sympathise. Indeed, the therapist may feel angry and frustrated towards the patient who seems both resistant and ungrateful.

THE TREATMENT OF CHOICE FOR TYPE 2 (COGNITIVE BEHAVIOURAL CONVERSION)

Having confidently diagnosed a psychogenic Type 2 dysphonia, the speech and language therapist needs to consider an appropriate therapeutic treatment approach. The decision to treat a Type 2 patient with traditional, symptomatic voice therapy techniques focusing on the body and voice and/or psychological methods, is largely determined by the weighting and complexity of predisposing and precipitating psychological factors within the history and their contribution to the maintenance of the voice disorder. However, as we cited earlier, we agree with Baker (2002) that a diagnosis of a psychogenic voice disorder implies 'that for true resolution, predisposing, precipitating and perpetuating psycho-emotional or psychosocial issues will need to be explored and addressed' (pp. 84–5). Perhaps the extent of the psychological therapeutic input versus the time given to symptomatic voice therapy will be influenced by the complexity of the predisposing, precipitating and perpetuating factors and of the insightfulness of the patient. We illustrate this in the case studies in Chapter 10.

Where a psychological approach is considered appropriate for the Type 2 group we would suggest cognitive behaviour therapy (CBT) as the treatment of choice since it is sympathetic to the Type 2 cognitive behavioural conversion features. Speech and language therapists also usually find this treatment modality is compatible with their own training background and enhances voice therapy. Collaboration in the workplace with a clinical psychologist skilled in CBT is an excellent way of accessing training. We have previously published examples of our work that illustrates both how using CBT with patients with a psychogenic dysphonia has led to improvements in both the inner conflict as well as the dysphonia in a group of patients who had been unresponsive to voice therapy alone, and have also illustrated how speech and language therapists can become more skilled and knowledgeable in psychological therapy through joint working with a clinical psychologist (Butcher et al. 1987; Butcher and Cavalli 1998).

THE TREATMENT OF CHOICE FOR PATIENTS WITH TYPE 3 (PSYCHOGENIC-HABITUATED)

Since the significant and precipitating stressful event or conflict will have diminished or resolved for this group, yet the patients will have developed a habituated faulty vocal muscle set, they are likely to respond well to symptomatic voice therapy. This approach, for treating both aphonics and dysphonics is detailed in Chapter 5.

There may be some value in including a degree of psychological therapy for these patients as a preventative measure to avoid recurrence. We would suggest that cognitive behaviour therapy would offer a framework and strategies that would be sympathetic to the needs of these patients. This might involve providing an understanding of the precipitating factors, such as recognition of stressful life events and their interplay with emotional and physical responses, and some exploration of predisposing factors such as the patient's rules for living and difficulty with self-expression. Psychological therapy for these patients is likely to be brief and will aim to provide understanding and closure of the original voice disorder as well as reducing the likelihood of recurrence. The SLT is well placed to provide this therapy, alongside symptomatic voice therapy, with a level of clinical supervision for a novice in this work.

THE TREATMENT OF CHOICE FOR PATIENTS WITH TRAUMA CONVERSION

The group that has its origin in an early or previous traumatic experience is more likely to respond to a combination of symptomatic voice therapy and psychological therapy. These patients will usually require input from someone experienced in psychotherapy and the course of treatment might well be extensive. However, if the therapist and patient can unearth and establish the link between the traumatic event and the PVD, a resolution is likely. These cases have not been widely reported or studied but the encouraging and thoughtful work from Baker (2003) provides helpful guidelines when thinking about and working with these patients. It highlights how important it is to consider not only whether there has been a trauma to the throat or voice or breathing in the near or distant past from which the person is now dissociated, but also to consider whether something has more recently reawakened the original trauma and triggered a conversion reaction in the form of PVD.

CLINICAL SUPERVISION

In the following chapter we describe the framework of cognitive behaviour therapy. We anticipate that speech and language therapists will find that both the structure of CBT, as well as the essential counselling skills required, fit comfortably with the way that voice therapists work. Nevertheless, although behaviour modification principles/ theory are taught to undergraduate speech and language therapists, CBT is not.

First of all, before embarking on CBT, we would recommend that the speech and language therapist had at least trained to have competencies in basic counselling skills. Indeed we would expect all speech and language therapists working in the field of voice to have these.

Second, once the speech and language therapist has chosen to use CBT and to employ the treatment strategies we would suggest that there are options of clinical supervision that the SLT should consider. In all cases we advocate that best practice requires the speech and language therapist to have regular supervision from a clinical psychologist or CBT specialist, wherein the therapist becomes familiar with the framework, the method of assessment and the various treatment strategies. As mentioned earlier, we have found that a model of co-working within therapy sessions is particularly beneficial in skilling the SLT. However, this is unlikely to be a model available to most therapists. We also recommend that the speech and language therapist have access to a clinical psychologist during the management of complex cases with CBT. This should preferably be through regular one-to-one or group supervision sessions although once a degree of supervision and learning has occurred it could be maintained through telephone supervision.

SUMMARY

- Psychogenic voice disorders are described as a dysphonia or aphonia where the causative or perpetuating factors are largely psychological or emotional conflict. The voice problem may manifest itself with musculoskeletal tension and hyperkinetic behaviours and these may eventually give rise to laryngeal pathology, these being products or symptoms of the underlying psychological cause.

- It is helpful to consider different categories of psychogenic voice disorder. Two main types of conversion voice disorder are discussed; Type 1, Freudian hysterical conversion disorder, which is rare (about 5%) and Type 2, a much more common conversion disorder (95%) that is closely linked to anxiety and where the locus of the precipitating conflict is closely associated with expression of feelings.

- The different types of conversion, Type 1 being *repression* and Type 2 being *suppression*, represent different coping mechanisms employed by the patient in the face of emotional conflict. Although each group of patients will have a predisposition to psychological problems as a result of life experiences and traumas, it is the personality type that will importantly influence their coping strategy and type of conversion.

- There is evidence that in some cases severe and persistent psychogenic dysphonia may eventually be traced back to a major traumatic stress experience associated with the voice or throat. In some cases of earlier traumatic experience the individual appears to cope with the experience through dissociation and the conversion reaction occurs either at the time of the original trauma or at a later date when an event briefly reawakens memories and emotions connected with the trauma. Because of the dissociated state, it is difficult for the patient and therapist to access and process the painful memories of the trauma, thus making therapy difficult.

- Furthermore, SLTs should recognise a Type 3 Psychogenic-Habituated voice disorder. Originally the person acquires an aphonia or dysphonia as a result of a psychogenic Type 2 aetiology, but in these cases the precipitating stressors or conflicts have diminished yet the person has developed a faulty vocal muscle set that has become habituated, thus prolonging the voice disorder. These patients respond primarily to a symptomatic voice therapy approach, although there may be some merit in providing brief psychological therapy in order to help the patient to understand the original conversion voice disorder and to prevent a recurrence.

- These three types of psychogenic voice disorders are distinct from a muscle misuse voice disorder that develops in the absence of significant psychological conflict or stress.

- To diagnose a psychogenic conversion voice disorder it is necessary not only to *exclude* significant laryngeal or neurological pathology, but also to positively *include a psychological aetiology.*
- Common aetiological features are discussed (pages 3–6) and these are categorised as Types 1 or 2 conversion (pages 10–15).
- The application of cognitive behaviour therapy (CBT) within the context of solid clinical supervision is recommended for the SLT when treating a Type 2 psychogenic conversion voice disorder.
- An understanding of the Types 1, 2 and 3 classification is useful because it helps the SLT identify some of the psychological processes operating. It also helps indicate which patients may be responsive to therapy and suggests why a minority are resistant to therapy of all persuasions. Finally, this classification helps the therapist determine when a symptomatic versus psychological therapeutic approach is best, e.g. a high number of presenting features of Type 2 may make CBT the treatment of choice.

2 Introducing the Cognitive Behaviour Therapy Model

In the previous chapter we introduced the reader to a new model of psychogenic voice disorder. Our intention was to present an approach that we hope will be helpful when trying to assess or make diagnostic sense of voice conditions that are primarily psychological in origin. In this chapter we want to introduce the reader to a particular psychological approach that we feel will enhance the speech and language therapist's range of skills when assessing and treating Type 2 psychogenic voice disorders. We are referring here to cognitive behaviour therapy.

THE ESSENCE OF COGNITIVE BEHAVIOUR THERAPY

In an earlier book (Butcher, Elias and Raven 1993) we began our introduction to cognitive behaviour therapy (CBT) by stressing its focus on phenomenology, self-awareness and self-education. We cited Davison and Neale's (1978) definition of **phenomenology** as '. . . the view that the phenomena of subjective experience should be studied because behaviour is considered to be determined by how the subject perceives himself and the world . . .' (p.648). We also cited Nordby and Hall's (1974) valuable emphasis that phenomenology is 'the description of the contents of immediate awareness, what is going on in a person's mind right now' (p.23–4). This emphasis is important in CBT because the therapist is concerned primarily with understanding the inner world of the person entering therapy and wants to know how the patient makes sense of experiences as well as how cognitions (thoughts and images) affect both emotions and behaviour. Since understanding this inner world requires self-awareness or the skill of self-monitoring on the part of the patient, a major focus in treatment is helping the individual increase awareness of thoughts and feelings in the day-to-day activities that occur between therapeutic meetings. In this way CBT also becomes a self-educational process through which increased self-knowledge provides the possibility of, or the potential for, personal change and development. To achieve these aims, cognitive behaviour therapists encourage self-observation on a daily basis and employ diary and record keeping and regular target setting in order to help individuals observe, record and change cognitive processes as well as emotional and behavioural reactions.

The next thing to appreciate about cognitive behaviour therapy is its holistic way of understanding human beings. As an approach, it casts a broad net that takes account of how emotional, psychosocial and biophysical processes shape behaviour. As suggested above, this holistic approach is grounded in recognising the important role of information processing or the ways in which the mind, or the person's thinking, deals with the information received from the inner and outer world of experiences.

In considering the essence of CBT the following should also be stressed:

- CBT is *an evolving discipline*, willing and able to incorporate views and methods that are consistent with its general systems theory principles and based on sound research evidence.
- All forms of CBT tend to be present- and target-centred, practical, structured and systematic in their approach to problem solutions.
- CBT is probably unique among the psychotherapies in always attempting, through regular summaries and feedback in sessions, to offer the client a clear explanation for their symptoms and a rationale for particular treatment strategies.

WHAT YOU WILL NEED TO KNOW

To start with, you will need to be introduced to the basic principles of this psychological model. Next, you will need to be well informed about skills and common therapeutic strategies which are needed in order to be proficient in this form of therapy. Then, you will need practice and supervision in order to become proficient as a cognitive behaviour therapist.

THE COGNITIVE ELEMENT OF THE THERAPY MODEL

While cognitive behaviour therapists do not assume that all behavioural change involves elaborate cognitive processes, they do assume that these processes commonly have a major influence on emotional, physical and behavioural states. They also assume that a great deal of mental processing is done automatically outside of conscious awareness. Take, for example, the way we process the following:

(i) John was on his way to school.
(ii) He was terribly worried about the maths lesson.
(iii) He thought he might not be able to control the class again today.
(iv) It was not a normal part of a janitor's duty.

(Cited in Williams et al. 1988, p.94)

Without questioning it most people immediately conclude from the first two sentences that John is a schoolboy having trouble with his maths. On digesting the third sentence they realise that this is not the case. However, they immediately assume John is a schoolteacher. The final sentence reveals that this too is an error!

Many psychologists take the view that in order for us to process data as quickly as we do, there must be relatively permanent structures in our memory (known as **schemas**) that are activated or triggered when stimulated by certain pieces of information. For example, information about someone on his way to school who was worrying about a maths lesson will trigger a 'schoolboy' or 'student' schema; the additional information that he is thinking, 'he might not be able to control the class', requires a re-evaluation of the 'schoolboy' schema (which now seems absurd or unbelievable) and triggers a 'schoolteacher' schema in order to give meaning to the additional information. However, the final sentence triggers a new schema. What we can note from this example is just how easily we make errors when automatically processing even simple sets of information.

A basic assumption or tenet in CBT is that specific types of errors in information processing have been formed sometime in the individual's past, probably, though not necessarily, at a very early age. These errors in thinking have become automatic, habitual responses to specific triggers and are the cause of many emotional and behavioural disturbances. Interestingly, research has shown that mood state is an important variable in shaping our thoughts. For example, people become more prone to negative, erroneous, irrational patterns of thinking when their mood is low or they are feeling depressed. It suggests that negative schemas might lie dormant until feeling emotionally low brings them to life. Whatever the explanation, and although we may disagree on how these schemas are formed and why they become active, we can at least say that a predominant pattern of negative thinking emerges in the context of lowered mood and declines once the mood has lifted. (See Segal et al. 2002, for a helpful discussion of these issues.)

Many cognitive therapists suggest that schemas are best seen as 'absolutes' or core beliefs that are triggered by life events. Because they are largely unconscious, schemas are not easily accessible. However, what we might observe if we look closely are underlying assumptions or beliefs in the form of internalised, cross-situational rules like 'If such-and-such, then so-and so'. As these guidelines in life can often be rather abstract, however, it is easy to miss their influence on our thinking and behaviour. What are most easily observable are the automatic thoughts (the 'internal commentaries') that arise from the schemas and underlying beliefs. How these different layers of thought affect our emotions and our behaviour is illustrated below:

Stimulus	Thought arising from a schema or underlying belief	Emotion arising from schema	Behaviour arising from schema
A man fails his driving test.	(Schema or belief about meaning of failure.) This shows I can't do this.	Anxiety	Does not try again
A wife sees her husband talking with an attractive woman from work.	(Schema about attractiveness/ desirability.) He's having an affair.	Suspicion/jealousy	Looking for clues; checking his activities
A crowded lift causes a man to have a panic attack.	(Schema about being trapped.) I can't cope with enclosed spaces.	Fear	Avoidance of enclosed spaces

(continued)

(*continued*)

A man experiences recurrent heart-burn.	(Schemas/beliefs about symptoms, illness, vulnerability.) I've got a heart condition.	Fear/depression	Repeatedly checking pulse; decreased physical exercise
A teenager is rejected by his girlfriend.	(Schemas/beliefs about the meaning of rejection.) If she doesn't love me I am unlovable and no one will ever love me. I have nothing to live for.	Depression	Attempted suicide
A man fails a job interview.	(Schemas/beliefs about meaning of failure, self-esteem.) I never do well at anything. No one will ever employ me.	Depression	Gives up making job applications
A woman is criticised by her husband and finds she cannot speak.	(Schemas/beliefs about male/female roles.) A woman should *never* shout at her husband. My husband is always right. I must never show my emotions.	Anger/frustration	Compliance, pleasing/ appeasing/ unassertiveness
A daughter is told by her mother that she is old enough to get her own accommodation.	(Schemas about self.) I cannot look after myself. I need other people for support.	Anxiety	Dependency, stubborn refusal to make change
A lump in the throat.	(Schemas about the meaning of physical symptoms.) I've got throat cancer.	Panic/depression	Seeking but not accepting reassurance
A teenager meeting an acquaintance.	(Schema about social skills.) I don't have anything to talk about.	Nervousness	Stammer, poor eye contact, agitation
A father is at times critical of his child for not doing homework.	(Schema about fairness.) He *never* says I do *anything* right.	Anger	Throwing toys, sulking, being oppositional

TEMPERAMENT AND LIFE EXPERIENCES

It is usually assumed that inherited temperamental characteristics play some part in the development of particular schemas. For example, a child who is easily startled as well as naturally shy and fearful of new situations and people will associate anxiety with these situations; exposure to these challenges would be expected to provoke or stimulate anxiety schemas. If, in addition, the child is exposed to traumatic life experiences such as maternal deprivation, physical abuse and parental rejection, this will not only reinforce the anxiety schemas associated with new experiences and people but will very likely produce personal schemas and underlying beliefs associated with being valueless, unlovable and inadequate. However, by contrast, in a supportive environment a nervous child can gain confidence through parental encouragement and through various successes so that new things are then construed schematically as 'challenging but not terrifying'.

Thus, an important part of the cognitive behavioural model is that temperamental *and* experiential factors shape the schemas we form about ourselves and our world. Therapeutically, therefore, accessing and exploring factors that may have predisposed the individual to develop certain types of schemas or underlying beliefs, is considered a central aspect of the cognitive behavioural approach. Some of the data connected with the above can be gathered through conventional history taking. However, to uncover schemas and to gain details of the individual's current thinking, therapists employ a technique known as Socratic Questioning or Socratic Communication, use formal questionnaires (e.g. the Schema Questionnaire, the Dysfunctional Attitude Scale), train clients in self-observation skills and ask them to keep daily record sheets of situations which provoke specific thoughts. (See Chapter 3.)

PREDISPOSING, PRECIPITATING AND PERPETUATING FACTORS (THE 3 Ps)

In terms of conducting a cognitive behavioural assessment of the presenting problem such as voice loss, an important guideline would be to consider factors such as temperament, life experiences, cognitions, biophysical and behavioural processes in terms of how they might *predispose, precipitate* or *perpetuate* voice change. For example, predisposing factors in the individual's dysphonia might be an introverted, shy, unassertive temperament, a dominating, authoritarian father, and harsh family rules discouraging personal expression of feelings. The precipitating factor might be an important or fundamental disagreement with her partner that she fears expressing because of her temperament and childhood learning, and the fear causes musculoskeletal tension affecting her voice. The perpetuating factors that might emerge over time could come from her ongoing frustration with not being able to challenge her partner, the continued inhibiting belief that she doesn't have a right to express her feelings, the conditioned response or habit of muscular tension, and habitual avoidance behaviour.

Another way of conceiving this process of change taking place over a short time span is to consider it in terms of what has been called the ABCs of cognitive behaviour therapy. The ABCs refer to the *Antecedent*, the **Belief** or **Behaviour** and the *Consequences* of that belief or behaviour. The therapist tries to understand what happened, the person's interpretation of the event(s), how he or she behaved, and the consequences of the belief and behaviour.

BIOPHYSICAL AND BEHAVIOURAL FACTORS

In recognising the influence of behavioural and biophysical features in the maintenance of individual problems, a cognitive behavioural model also assumes that these factors need to be fully assessed. For example, particularly in stress-related or anxiety disorders like psychogenic voice loss, it will always be necessary to consider the presence of such things as musculoskeletal tension, autonomic arousal, hyperventilation, fight-or-flight reactions, and any classical and operant conditioning which may be maintaining certain patterns of behaviour. Consideration of these features and approaches to treatment are given in Chapters 6 and 7.

MULTIPLE TREATMENT STRATEGIES

Finally, the CBT model assumes that if all these factors are taken into consideration, it is possible to develop treatment strategies that will create positive change in thoughts, emotions, and physical and behavioural reactions. In targeting changes in these areas, CBT attempts to be comprehensive in intervention and to employ multiple treatment strategies to treat individual problems. Thus, for example, someone with an anxiety state may be taught stress management techniques involving a variety of cognitive, physical, behavioural strategies and taken through a course of graded, *in vivo* desensitisation.

The features of the cognitive behavioural model outlined above also need to be integrated with a number of skills that are a necessary part of practising CBT.

A KNOWLEDGE OF PSYCHOPATHOLOGY

The therapist must be able to recognise serious psychopathological states that may be resistant to CBT or where a referral to another specialist may be necessary. In particular, the therapist needs to distinguish the anxiety and mild depressive states, which are common to voice disorders, from more serious psychopathology. These more difficult to treat conditions include:

- some anxiety disorders like panic disorder and obsessive-compulsive disorder
- mania
- clinical depression or major depressive disorder
- some types of somatoform disorder
- personality disorder and
- schizophrenia.

While it will be quite rare to encounter these conditions in a voice clinic, we have on occasions assessed patients with functional voice problems who fit a diagnosis of, for example, personality disorder, phobic anxiety disorder and post-traumatic anxiety disorder. To help you know what to look for and when to think about a referral to an appropriate specialist, we will give a detailed description of these psychological disorders in Chapter 9.

COGNITIVE BEHAVIOUR THERAPIST SKILLS

Butcher and Elias (1994) suggest that apart from familiarity with the theoretical model, the practice of cognitive behaviour therapy requires skills that can be summarised in the following table:

Table 2.1: Basic guidelines and essential skills in cognitive-behaviour therapy

The therapist needs skill in:
1. creating a sound therapeutic relationship
2. thinking holistically and systematically about psychological processes
3. using various forms of data collection, e.g. standard history, questionnaires, daily record sheets
4. formulating tentative hypotheses for testing in treatment
5. making the treatment model explicit
6. giving feedback on findings and formulations
7. highlighting the role of collaboration and self-help
8. providing a clear plan of action, description of aims, treatment contract, etc.

In the following chapter you will find these essential skills described in detail for your guidance.

COGNITIVE BEHAVIOURAL TREATMENT STRATEGIES

For speech and language therapists working with voice, we consider the most important cognitive behavioural strategies to be as follows:

1   assessing the client's thinking
2   highlighting and changing dysfunctional thoughts
3   teaching stress management strategies
4   assessing and treating depressive symptoms caused by stress
5   training clients in communication and social interaction skills
6   training clients in life management skills

(Butcher 1994)

These broad treatment strategies will be explored in detail and also illustrated through various case study examples in Chapters 6, 7, 8 and 10.

SUMMARY

To summarise this brief introduction to CBT principles, therapist skills and treatment strategies, and as an aid to learning and ease of reference, we conclude with a check list of factors highlighted in the preceding section.

Check list of cognitive behaviour therapy principles:

- holistic and integrative approach
- assumption that schemas play a role in dysfunctional thinking, feeling and behaviour
- assessment of individual differences, life experiences and the 3 Ps
- consideration of behavioural and biophysical features
- development of (often multiple) forms of data collection
- target-specific treatment strategies.

Check list of cognitive behaviour therapist skills:

- creating a sound therapeutic relationship
- thinking holistically and systematically about psychological processes
- using various forms of data collection, e.g. standard history, questionnaires, daily record sheets
- formulating tentative hypotheses for testing in treatment
- making the treatment model explicit
- giving feedback on findings and formulations
- highlighting the role of collaboration and self-help
- providing a clear plan of action, description of aims, treatment contract, etc.
- (Further elaboration of these skills is provided in Chapter 3.)
- awareness of therapeutic limits. The therapist is reminded of the need to recognise serious psychological states and to consider referral to an appropriate specialist. Detailed description and management guidance will be given in Chapter 9.

Check list of cognitive behavioural treatment strategies:

- assessing the client's thinking
- highlighting and changing dysfunctional thoughts
- teaching stress management strategies
- assessing and treating depressive symptoms caused by stress
- training clients in communication and social interaction skills
- training clients in life management skills.

3 Cognitive Behaviour Therapy: Essential Assessment Principles and Therapist Skills

This chapter will attempt to detail the basic skills underpinning cognitive behaviour therapy. Most readers will be familiar with many of these skills and use them regularly in their work. However, it must be emphasised that a person is practising cognitive behaviour therapy only when these different skills are consistently and systematically integrated into a particular style of working. To reach this point, the voice therapist should have had some formal training and supervision from a therapist experienced in CBT.

From the beginning of treatment, the cognitive behaviour therapist should be employing the skills summarised in Table 2.1, p. 37. For the novice therapist this summary probably needs some elaboration.

CREATING A SOUND THERAPEUTIC RELATIONSHIP

Creating a sound therapeutic relationship – establishing a rapport and putting the client at ease in what they may feel is a worrying or threatening situation – is important in most professions involved in the assessment and treatment of individual medical or personal problems. The atmosphere must enable clients to talk openly, honestly and freely about their private and personal life; they must feel that their revelations will be held in confidence and that these will be treated sympathetically or uncritically. Clients must also feel that the therapist not only shows empathy and warmth but that these responses are genuine. Finally, clients have to feel convinced that the therapist understands what they are trying to articulate or communicate. Research has suggested (see Rogers 1961) that the most important therapist qualities in these areas include the following triad:

- unconditional warmth or regard
- empathy
- genuineness.

THINKING HOLISTICALLY AND SYSTEMATICALLY

As suggested earlier, CBT emphasises the information processing role of mental activities and the effect this has on emotions and behaviour. More than this, however,

CBT recognises the importance of systematically assessing the individual's social, developmental, emotional experiences, the way behaviour may be classically and operantly conditioned and the individual differences in how these events are construed subjectively. Essentially, a cognitive behavioural assessment should take account of the following categories and should recognise and understand the types of influence each may have on the other:

- genetic/biological features (inherited predispositions in temperament and personality)
- environmental factors
- developmental experiences, life events
- interpersonal relationships
- cognitions (thoughts *and* imagery)
- affect or emotions
- physiological reactions (e.g. autonomic arousal, musculoskeletal tension)
- behavioural responses, classical and operant conditioning, habituation, generalisation.

In taking account of these existential, social and psychophysical processes, the therapist must also recognise the sort of influence each may have on the other. For example, in a person who, temperamentally, has inherited a sensitive or labile nervous constitution, a fearful thought such as 'I haven't studied enough to pass this exam,' may produce an anxiety state with significant physiological, behavioural and cognitive reactions (diarrhoea, vomiting, restlessness, sleeplessness, distractibility, problems with studying). In a student with a more robust constitution the same thought would very likely produce some anxiety but, because it is less overwhelming, this might foster greater motivation, longer hours of study, more focused concentration and a sense of progress or achievement, as well as positive feelings that in themselves further promote motivation and restful sleep.

In thinking about the assessment you may find it helpful to refer to **the 3 Ps** (the predisposing, the precipitating and perpetuating factors) and **the ABCs** (the antecedent event, the belief and behaviour and the consequences of that belief or behaviour) described in Chapter 2, p. 35–6.

INDIVIDUAL DIFFERENCES

The examples above also illustrate how the therapist is taking account of individual differences or the uniqueness of the individual case. The individual difference noted so far between our two students was the difference between a labile and a stable nervous system and the consequences emotionally and behaviourally. We might predict that the first student will fail his exams and, as a consequence of the whole experience, develop a phobia of studying and examinations, while the second student's motivation and hard work pays off, he catches up on his work and passes with flying colours. However, not only are individual differences more complex than this but other factors may need to be considered such as, for example, interpersonal relationships. Supposing our first student has a close friend who invites him to join a revision group to help catch up with work and also suggests joining a yoga class and taking up jogging together to help with relaxation. This social support and encouragement from the friend combined with the practical self-help strategy of the revision group improve his confidence about passing the exams. The yoga and physical exercise not only help him relax but in combination with his improved confidence, have a direct positive effect on concentration and getting off to sleep.

In contrast, past and current relationships in the life of our second student begin to hamper his progress in revision. From a very early age, his parents have always demanded excellence in academic pursuits. Although he is catching up on his work, he begins to fear he will not live up to these expectations. This thought causes some anxiety and some sleepless nights but his concentration is still good and he continues to work hard. However, about a week before his exams, he discovers that his girlfriend, with whom he is deeply emotionally involved, is two-timing with his best friend. Not only is this a complete surprise but he is particularly shocked because of the high ideals he holds about friendship and loyalty. Furthermore, he is someone who has had difficulty being trustful of others in relationships and for the first time had lowered his defences and allowed himself to become deeply involved with a woman. In the emotional turmoil that follows he finds it impossible to keep his mind on revision and becomes more and more panic-stricken about passing his exams and living up to the demands of his parents. On the day of the first exam he has a panic attack and rushes from the room – an experience and action which conditions phobic avoidance behaviour in relation to all other exams in the following week, thus leaving him with a major obstacle in relation to completing his studies. Student 1 with exam stress has a labile nervous system (which means he's easily made anxious) but social support, positive thinking and exercise, etc., reduce his anxiety and he passes his exam.

Example in Summary

Using an ABC analysis might suggest the following process as a way of understanding Student 1: Realisation of the closeness of his exam and amount of work not done (the *Antecedent event*) triggers the *Belief,* 'I haven't studied enough to pass my exam,' as well as *Behavioural* change, and the *Consequences* are an anxiety state and distractibility, etc. For Student 2 the *Antecedent* event is the disloyalty of his friend and girlfriend that evokes the *Belief,* 'People you trust must always be loyal,' the associated *Behavioural* change, and the *Consequent* mental confusion and emotional turmoil.

In using a 3 Ps analysis with Student 1 you would consider his sensitive or labile nervous system as a *Predisposing* factor, that his anxiety is *Precipitated* by the approach of his exam and his belief about not being prepared, and the anxiety is

Perpetuated by, for example, his distractibility confirming his belief about not doing enough work. For Student 2 you might consider that his belief about the importance of loyalty *Predisposes* him to anxiety in the event that people he is close to fail to meet expectations. The anxiety is *Precipitated* by the disloyal behaviour of both friend and girlfriend and *Perpetuated* by an unresolved mental and emotional turmoil.

By illustrating the individual personal life experiences of two people faced with the challenge of passing an examination, we hope to have illustrated the sort of understanding and consideration that is needed in making a cognitive behavioural assessment. Assessing individual differences and psychological processes while at the same time attempting to achieve a complete picture – through seeing how one process influences another – is a core skill in cognitive behavioural assessment, formulation and treatment development. Because processes are complex and they interact one with another, the formulation leads quite naturally to the use of multiple treatment strategies rather than a one-dimensional focus. However, before this can be thought about, the therapist must be familiar with a variety of ways of making sure the assessment is fully comprehensive. (See Chapter 10 for examples of 3 Ps.)

USING VARIOUS FORMS OF DATA COLLECTION

We get a good idea of *what* information we need to gather and in *which* areas we need to focus from the list of eight social, psychological, biophysical, and behavioural factors on page 40. However, we need to know *how* to collect data about these categories. The data collected must help the therapist form a picture of where problems originate as well as the influence this has on particular processes like thoughts and feelings. It should also indicate which treatment strategies are more likely to be beneficial. This requires good interviewing and history taking skills as well as skill in other forms of information gathering such as standard questionnaires and use of daily record sheets.

QUESTIONNAIRES

Questionnaires provide a formal, structured and standardised means of assessment. They can be helpful as screening devices and for covering factors that need to be considered in a formulation. The Irritability-Depression-Anxiety Scale, (Snaith et al. 1978), the Hospital Anxiety and Depression Scale (HADS) (Zigmond and Snaith 1983), the Beck Depression Inventory (Beck and Steer 1987) and the Beck Anxiety Inventory (Beck and Steer 1990) can be cited as examples of questionnaires that are helpful screening and diagnostic tools. However, a CBT assessment involves more than diagnosing or categorising psychological symptoms. To get beyond symptoms and to assess underlying thoughts and schemas, questionnaires like the Dysfunctional Attitude Scale (DAS) (Burns 1980) and the Young Schema Questionnaire (Young and Brown 2003) might be employed. These give an indication of the dysfunctional thinking patterns that either emerge in association with mood disturbance or are themselves the cause of anxiety and depression. Therefore, questionnaires can provide helpful information about symptomatology, offer a guide to the type of psychological condition and suggest underlying features and causes. Many of these questionnaires can be completed within a few minutes. In the case of the HADS and Burns (1980) adaptation of the DAS, clients can complete the questionnaire in their own time and score it for themselves. Questionnaires do not need to be given routinely but are most usefully employed when trying to answer specific questions about underlying psychological features or processes.

REFLECTING

In reflecting, the interviewer or therapist rephrases something the client has mentioned. This helps the patient to reconsider what they have said and to clarify their thoughts. Through reflecting, the therapist also conveys that he or she is listening and understanding what was said, thus fostering rapport, and it frequently elicits additional, often important, information from the client:

> **Client:** I was arguing with my daughter and she got angry and started shouting at me. I went to reply and nothing came out.
> **Therapist:** She got angry and you couldn't speak?
> **Client:** Yes. This had never happened before with her. But then we were fighting over a big issue to do with how much freedom she should have now that she's 17. She was very determined to have her way.
> **Therapist:** Then, if I understand this correctly, the first time you lost your voice with your daughter was when she got angry over the limits you were setting and when she was questioning your authority?
> **Client:** That's right. I suppose I've never liked being authoritarian with her. Whenever I'm strict, she resents it and can make me feel she doesn't love me, which I find is very hurtful. So I tend to let her have her way and don't say anything. Everyone says she's spoilt and I think they're probably right. I just can't stand getting into a fight with her though and then feeling she doesn't love me. That's why I won't say anything. In case she gets upset. This time, however, I thought it was really important. I really had to say something and that's when I found I couldn't.

By thoughtfully reflecting back the client's statements, the interviewer has gathered important information about the dynamics of a troubled relationship between a mother and daughter. The new information suggests there may be a link between the mother's emotional conflict over expressing or enforcing views and her voice loss. This may prompt the interviewer to enquire about other occasions in which expressing feeling has been difficult and also whether these occasions affect voice production.

Therapeutically, reflection can also be a valuable way of summing up possible causes of problems and, through doing this, may provide the client with an interpretation that helps them understand their difficulties. Thus, the therapist might reflect at the end of this session: 'From what you were saying today about finding it difficult to set limits with your daughter, it seems that if you try to be strict she has a way of making you feel unloved and hurt. To avoid this you usually let her have her way but when it was really important, when there was a lot at stake, and you tried to stand up to her, your voice let you down.'

LISTENING

In describing the importance of reflection as an assessment and therapeutic skill, it was indicated that listening attentively to what the client describes is essential. While receptive listening is an important skill in any interview setting, cognitive behavioural interviewing requires more than just the registering and recording of facts. The interviewer needs to be alert to hidden messages or implicit meanings in what is being described and to be able to make intuitive connections that can then be evaluated or tested through further questioning. As illustrated above, the client's description of her conflict with her daughter suggested a connection between voice loss and conflict over expressing feelings or asserting herself through setting limits. In addition, a cognitive behaviour therapist would speculate about other psychosocial processes going on in the relationship that may be important. For instance, the information gathered so far should prompt the following questions:

- What does your daughter *actually* do when she gets angry?
- How do you know she is determined to have her way? How does she *show* this?
- How does she make you feel she doesn't love you?
- When you say it is 'hurtful' what do you mean? How does it *feel*? What do people *mean* when they say your daughter is spoilt? Can you *define* this? What do *you* mean when you say your daughter is spoilt?
- What do you mean when you say you 'can't stand' getting into a conflict with her?
- Why was it so important you say something on this particular occasion?
- What *effect* do you think it has on your daughter when you always let her have her own way?
- What do you think she thinks of you at these times?

In asking these questions, the interviewer is using his or her knowledge of the CBT model to explore ways in which certain cognitive and behavioural patterns or processes may be established and manifest. Answers to these questions will build up a more detailed, whole picture. Notice too how comprehensive the questioning is, covering **cognitive**, **emotional** and **behavioural** features.

OBSERVING AND QUESTIONING

In terms of non-verbal communication from the client, listening also includes being aware of changes in voice quality, breathing patterns and body posture. Qualitative changes in voice when the client touches on certain topics may be important psychologically. It will usually indicate strong emotions attached to the topic and suggest issues that will have to be addressed in therapy.

We can also gather additional information about the client from observing aspects of behaviour. For example, downcast countenance, lifeless eyes or tearfulness and flattened affect are reliable indicators of depression; poor eye contact and hesitant speech will suggest shyness or lack of social confidence; while agitation or restlessness, muscular tension, perspiration and rapid, shallow breathing, are symptoms associated with an anxiety state. (Obviously, these interpretations have assumed the therapist has previously excluded any medical/organic causation of such symptoms.)

There may be times during the interview and later in treatment when touching on a certain topic triggers not only changes in voice quality but hesitation in speech, facial tension, a moistening of the eyes, shifts of posture or fidgeting. Any one or combination of these indicators of troubled thoughts and painful emotions will alert the interviewer and provide an opportunity for asking further questions. Quite often at these moments, a sensitive question will not only convey empathy but can produce information which is critical in gaining a full understanding of problem areas.

- That appeared to be quite hard to talk about. . .?
- I noticed you looked quite sad as you were talking and I wondered what was going through your mind. . . ?
- You looked a little troubled when you mentioned that. . . ?
- I was wondering what you were thinking about just then. . .?
- You seemed to get quite tense when I asked you about your mother and I wondered what your thoughts were. . .?

THE BASICS OF ASKING GOOD QUESTIONS

The first rule of good interviewing is remembering to keep the questions short, simple and jargon-free. The second rule is to avoid too many 'closed questions' or questions to which a person can respond with a 'yes' or a 'no' and which may pre-empt elaboration or influence the reply. For example, 'Although you had a voice problem, were you pleased to be starting work?' 'Did you get on okay with your work colleagues?' 'Was your boss helpful?'

It is much better to use 'open questions,' which require a considered, elaborated response in the person's own words. For example, 'Given that you had a voice problem, how did it feel to be starting work?' 'What did you think of your colleagues?' 'How would you describe your boss?' Open questions will add depth or fill in important gaps in the overall picture. For example, 'What do you recall about the first time you had a voice problem?' 'How did it *feel*?' 'What was it like?' 'How did it seem at the time?' 'How did your voice problem affect your job?' 'What did you think was wrong?'

If a reply to an open question does not give as much information as required, a good interviewer can use a combination of open and closed questions to good effect.

Interviewer: What were you feeling when you thought about confronting your husband?

Client: Anxious.

Interviewer: What was that like?

Client: Churning in my stomach. Sweating. Tense. Dry mouth.

Interviewer: Anything else?

Client: Not that I recall.

Interviewer: Was your heart racing?

Client: Yes, it certainly was.

Interviewer: Did you notice whether you were breathing differently?

Client: No. Wait a minute. It became very rapid – like I needed more air or something.

(Butcher, Elias and Raven 1993, p.54)

SOCRATIC QUESTIONS AND SOCRATIC DIALOGUE

Christine Padesky (2002) states that using Socratic questioning assumes that your client has the knowledge to provide the answer and that a Socratic dialogue with your client should have four stages: *Asking Informational Questions*; *Listening*; *Summarising*; and *Asking Analytical/Synthesising Questions*. These qualities of Socratic questioning are common to all forms of cognitive behaviour therapy. However, Padesky's summary is particularly helpful because it systematically describes how this form of data gathering not only provides important information for the therapist but encourages the client to think anew and to re-evaluate old assumptions about their problem:

Informational Questions

In asking informational questions the therapist will ask for *specific examples. Questions will cover Who? What? Where? When?* The interviewer will ask about the client's *emotional response*, enquire *in what way is this a problem* for the client, question *how they responded in the past* and *what they would confide to a friend*.

Listening

Padesky emphasises that good listening involves *responding positively verbally and non-verbally and using empathic reflections*. She suggests that for future reference the therapist should *note the client's use of words, images* or *metaphors*, and particular *ideas* or *beliefs* that describe their experience. She also stresses that in this process the therapist should *identify* both the client's *strengths* and their *apparent weaknesses*. Finally, someone skilled in listening is also alert for *things not being said, conscious or unconscious avoidance, uneasiness or difficulty revealing some things*.

Summarising

Padesky's style of summarising is to state the client's initial belief – where this is appropriate – and follow this with a concise summary of key information collected so far. She suggests that this is best done in writing a list of key points and shared with the client along with the suggestion that together they consider how the information could be valuable or helpful.

Asking Analytic/Synthesising Questions

We could sum up Padesky's description of asking analytic/synthesising questions as asking those questions that draw out *the client's view of their problem* and *what they think might help*. Here the therapist finds ways of asking the client 'How do you make sense of the difficulty you're having?' 'How do you think *this (belief/ experience)* goes with *that* (belief/experience)?' 'Have you any thoughts on what might help?' 'What would you tell a good friend about this?' 'What do you think they would say?' and so on. (See Christine Padesky 2002, p. 6 and also *www.padesky.com.*)

DOWNWARD ARROW TECHNIQUE

Downward arrow technique is a method of getting behind a statement to the underlying meaning of what is being said by asking questions that help the person define 'the thought behind the thought'. The method is frequently used to get at what is really disturbing the person and employs the following type of questions:

What would that mean to you?
How would that be a problem?
What would that say about you?
What would happen then?

The following example of downward arrow questioning is taken from a treatment session with a patient who was trying to understand her difficulty revealing how she feels to her boyfriend and her fear of reacting wrongly:

Reacting wrongly would be getting angry.
Why would that be so bad?
I'd be showing emotion.
And what would the emotion say?
You've hurt me.
What would be so bad about saying that?
It will be trodden on.
If your feelings were trodden on, what would that mean?
The feelings don't get the reaction they deserve. They're dismissed.
And why is that so bad?

It makes me feel I'm not worth anything. Like when I went to my father and said I'm frightened and he didn't like that.
And what does that mean to you?
That you don't love me anymore.
So, if you reveal your feelings, what happens then?
You will be judged.

A second example of downward arrow questioning is taken from a therapy session where the patient – a man who has never been able to please his overbearing mother – is trying to understand why he has been staying in and avoiding people.

Indoors I feel better protected.
So what does going outdoors mean to you?
I'm vulnerable.
In what way does going outdoors make you vulnerable?
It feels like someone's going to have a go at me.
If someone had a go at you, what would that mean?
I'm in the wrong.
In what way would you be in the wrong?
I don't fit in. I'm an oddity.
And why is that so bad?
I feel guilty. I'm not working. People would say you should be pulling your weight.
And if they said that, why would that be a problem?
People would discard me.
And what would that mean to you?
I must get it right. If I don't get it right, if I don't toe the line, people will have a go at me.

Through the downward arrow questions the therapist and patient uncover underlying assumptions or core beliefs that have not previously been made explicit or conscious.

CONSTRUCTIVE QUESTIONS AND LANGUAGE

A more recent development in CBT has been to emphasise the use of positive questions and language. Cognitive therapists have traditionally used what might be called **deconstructive** language and questioning to understand and treat specific problems. By contrast, the use of **constructive** questions and language focuses more on the present and future potential for positive change within the client. The shift in emphasis is away from having an entirely **problem focus** that sees changing the problem as the primary therapeutic goal to having a **possibility focus**, which aims to draw out the client's creative potential for positive change or personal growth. Christine Padesky (2002) has highlighted how constructive questions and language should be part of her four pillars of therapy described on pages 46–7.

Constructive Informational Questions

Constructive informational questions involve moving away from detailed questions about the problem to asking how the person would like things to change, how they would like to be, and what would have to occur for this to come about. It includes asking how that would feel and asking for specific examples.

Constructive Listening Tips

Padesky suggests that constructive listening involves (a) being alert to the presence of new or positive cognitions, behaviours and emotional responses as well as (b) using the core counselling skills of showing verbal and non-verbal interest to reinforce any constructive or creative suggestions or responses from the client.

Constructive Summaries

Constructive summaries involve summarising in a way that is both constructive and positive in the language you use. Examples would be, 'You want to be a more positive person' rather than saying, 'You've emphasised how negative you feel about things' or 'You'd like to socialise more' rather than 'You're sick of being stuck at home because you can't make yourself heard when you speak.'

Constructive Analytical/Synthesising Questions

By using constructive analytic/synthesising questions the therapist attempts to get the client to do some positive thinking about the problem. For example, asking the client to consider how certain things would improve life, how what has been summarised would make a positive difference or how these ideas or changes might be helpful in the current situation. (See Christine Padesky 2002, p.10 and also *www.padesky.com*.)

DAILY RECORD SHEETS

Objectivity, unambiguous or clear definitions, reliability, and replication in data collection, are distinguishing features in behavioural science. The development of behaviour therapy has always emphasised the importance of achieving high standards in these areas, and an innovation by cognitive therapists in recent times has been to adapt the behavioural methods of data collection in order to gather information about subjective processes. Whereas behaviour therapists regularly focused on selecting, observing and rating specific behaviours or sets of behaviours on record sheets for later analysis or quantification, the cognitive therapists encouraged their clients to make daily subjective observations of thoughts, images and emotions and to record these on specially designed record sheets. While the approach may be compared to keeping a diary, there is at least one significant difference: the diary keeping of subjective processes is structured so that the recording is done in a specific way, usually in columns with headings and usually starting with a record of an event or situation that preceded (or has been assumed to trigger) the particular thoughts, emotions and actions. The record sheet can be as simple as three columns headed The Situation, Your Thoughts, What You Did, or headed The Situation, Unhelpful Thoughts, Helpful Thoughts. By this means, the therapist is able to amass recent – hence, reasonably reliable – details of events which evoke specific cognitions as well as emotional and behavioural responses.

As therapy progresses, the daily record form can also be used as an aid to the therapeutic process. For example, the client can be asked to practise analysing the type of thinking error evoked by a specific event or situation and to consider ways that he or she could think more appropriately or rationally. For example, observing a situation provoking a self-critical thought, 'I never do anything right,' the client could categorise this as an overgeneralisation. He or she could then reason in the following way: 'Everyone makes mistakes. I shouldn't be so hard on myself and should think how often I don't make mistakes or do well at things,' etc., thus changing self-criticism into self-praise and doing something to change their emotional state from negative (e.g. anxious, low or depressed) to positive (e.g. calm, buoyant, accepting or satisfied).

A carefully designed daily record form used over a short period prior to treatment can also be a valuable means of obtaining a base line of situations, cognitions, behaviours and symptoms, thus giving an indication of their frequency and severity and providing a comparative yardstick when trying to measuring the effect of intervention. Examples of daily record sheets can be found in Chapters 6 and 8.

FORMULATING TENTATIVE HYPOTHESES

Another essential skill in cognitive behavioural interviewing and therapy is the ability to think in terms of explanations or hypotheses that, hopefully, will then be evaluated or tested through the programme of treatment. The definition of behaviour therapy as 'the experimental investigation of the individual case' (Yates 1970, p.19) also applies to cognitive behaviour therapy. This means that on formulating the view as to the causes of an individual problem, the therapist should approach intervention with a scientific attitude: testing out the hypothesis by developing a valid, reliable, clearly defined and systematic means of data collection, establishing a base-line period (for example, when assessing aphonia, finding a way of rating over a week or two the frequency of voice loss or recovery before beginning intervention), removing variables or influences which would distort or contaminate the results, and, finally, using appropriate methods to assess or rate the findings. The outcome of intervention or measure of changes should prove or disprove the hypothesis. For example, if we conclude that a patient's voice problem is caused by a fear of the consequences of expressing her views to her daughter, the therapist would predict that once the patient resolves this conflict, expresses her views and finds the consequences are not as bad as predicted, the voice will return to normal. If this does not happen as predicted, the hypothesis may have to be abandoned and replaced by an alternative explanation or more consideration given to additional factors inhibiting recovery. For example, your hypothesis might be right but the faulty mechanism of the voice may have habituated. Again, it may be that, currently, there are additional stressful events making an easy resolution more difficult and these factors may need further exploration in order to achieve a successful conclusion to therapy.

Methodologically, Yates (1970) had in mind a detailed individual case study with a base line and experimental conditions. However, because therapeutic intervention will usually be multifocused, and given that it is rarely possible in the clinical setting to be as rigorously scientific as one might like, this will not be an easy task. Despite these difficulties, the principles should guide all interventions and the therapist should take the trouble to gain a record of the circumstances in which the symptoms occur as well as their frequency and severity before commencing treatment.

QUESTIONS TO ASK YOURSELF

Given that the formulation provides tentative hypotheses that are tested through treatment, the therapist will have an open and non-rigid approach to the client's problems and to therapy. The therapist will be constantly evaluating progress, looking for support for their view and, perhaps more importantly, asking:

'Does this new bit of information cast a different light on how I've been viewing the main cause of this problem?'
'How could I "test" this?' 'How should I vary what I am already doing?' 'If my theory is right, why isn't this working? What have I missed?'
'How can I "test" whether this new way of looking at things is right?' etc.

Case example

The initial assessment (including daily ratings of circumstances, frequency and severity) of dysphonia in a female school teacher suggested the hypothesis that the prime factors maintaining her voice loss were largely environmental and behavioural – repeatedly raising her voice to control difficult, rowdy classes, regular duties in a noisy playground that required her to shout to be heard, some evenings running two hour adult education classes which involved almost constant talking above a noisy ventilation system, and regular socialising in crowded, smoky environments such as pubs and nightclubs which placed additional demand on her voice.

These features might suggest a treatment approach that involves behavioural strategies such as use of a voice abuse diary, a vocal rest programme and targets for changing the specific work and social behaviours that the therapist assumes are the cause of voice loss. However, when the patient's voice fails to improve with this treatment – having tested out the behavioural hypothesis – then the therapist should realise that other factors need consideration and that a re-formulation and new hypotheses are necessary.

Of course, abandoning the behavioural hypothesis does not mean that the behavioural features are unimportant. They may, in themselves, be making a major contribution to the voice loss. It simply means that the behavioural interpretation is too limited to provide a full explanation of why this individual has lost her voice. Therefore, the treatment outcome is likely to be more positive if one considers causal factors more comprehensively. The value of the behavioural intervention and testing this out through treatment has been to show that the first formulation or hypothesis is too simplistic or one dimensional and should either be abandoned or, as is commonly the case, developed into a more sophisticated formulation or hypothesis.

When questioned more closely the client admitted being caught up in an important inter-personal stress at school where she disagreed fundamentally with many of her head teacher's policies but felt unable to speak her mind because she feared she would alienate or anger him. Given the association between dysphonia, poor response to treatment, and difficulties expressing feelings (Butcher et al. 1987) or being caught in a 'conflict over speaking out' (House & Andrews 1988), we could hypothesise that the tension with her head teacher is an important cause in voice loss and that if this were addressed the voice would then improve. A number of cognitive behavioural techniques could be used as a means of testing out this possibility: recording and challenging negative thoughts about expressing views, training in positive self-instruction, practising assertion through role playing or trying out assertion in social situations which are only mildly threatening, stress management training, target setting, graded exposure, etc. Again, in this and any other case, outcome would help us accept or reject the hypothesis we are using.

PROVIDING THE CLIENT WITH A REVIEW OF YOUR THOUGHTS, FINDINGS AND FORMULATION

When problems are psychological in origin or where no medical or physical cause can be found, the majority of patients will be baffled by their symptoms. Being told that their problem is not physical is rarely reassuring. Patients often conclude that the doctor believes they are either imagining or causing the symptoms. Even if they consider a psychological cause, they may confuse themselves further with popular psychology. For example, with voice loss it is popularly held that symptoms of this sort may be an unconscious way of gaining attention that compensates for the inconvenience of not having a voice. An interpretation of this sort when it is not the case might be expected to make the sufferer feel not only baffled and helpless but humiliated and angry at the thought that this is what others think is going on. It is, therefore, important to deal with these issues, not only formulating an initial view of the factors causing and maintaining the loss of voice but conveying these in simple terms to the client. *In offering this, it is essential, first of all, to describe the relationship between stress and voice loss to the client.* It is assumed that helping the client make more sense of his or her problems not only reduces the mystification and its accompanying confusion, uncertainty and stress, but enables the client to make sense, and best use, of the CBT approach. This also leads to negotiation on what can be offered.

Typically, an explanation will begin at the end of the assessment with a summing up of what the therapist feels are important issues. Usually this will cover developmental and psychosocial experiences and recent life events, reference to the physical and psychological consequences of stress (for example, autonomic arousal, physical tension, anxiety) and how this is pertinent to the patient's current difficulties. Given the limited time the SLT has to conduct both an assessment of voice and a CBT assessment, the explanation will probably be quite brief in the first session. We will illustrate how best to do this in Chapter 4 and need only add here that the summary should conclude with the therapist checking the patient's response and by saying something like 'I don't know if this way of looking at things makes sense to you? Have I missed anything that feels important?'

In addition to this sort of summarising and checking for accuracy, it should be kept in mind that cognitive behaviour therapists repeatedly give summaries of what has been covered during the course of each therapy session. This might be done by saying 'From what you just said, am I right in thinking . . .' or, 'Are you saying that if [this] then [that]?' Better still, the therapist might see what conclusions the patient has reached by asking, 'How do you think [this] might relate to [that]?'

MAKING THE TREATMENT MODEL EXPLICIT

Providing a review of thoughts and findings in the first session can set the stage for talking in more detail about the CBT model (for example, describing the connection between thoughts, emotions and physical tension) and introducing, as well as justifying, specific treatment strategies (for example, anxiety management training and keeping daily records of situations and thoughts) when commencing treatment. Thus, in offering a formulation followed by a description of the therapeutic model, the therapist provides the patient with a way of understanding their experience, hence reducing confusion and anxiety, and giving a way of thinking about and working toward overcoming difficulties which should foster their motivation to change. The therapist might say the following:

'Because we believe that what we think has an impact on how we feel and behave, we'll be spending some time in our sessions together looking at the thoughts you have when you want to speak your mind. We'll ask you to keep a record in the week of when these situations arise. For example, we might find that when you go to speak to your boyfriend about what you want, you're thinking you don't have the right to question him or that he'll get angry, won't like you or might even leave you. If that's the case, I'd expect you to feel anxious, and the anxiety might stop you from speaking your mind. So the first thing we might do is question whether there's any reality in the worries you're having. For example, have you considered that instead of getting angry, your boyfriend might respect you more for having a view of your own? Thinking about the outcome in a more positive way should help you feel less anxious and make it a bit easier to speak to him. We'll also be looking at practical ways of reducing your anxiety and increasing your confidence in these situations. For example, you might find it helpful to learn some ways of keeping yourself physically relaxed at these times and to rehearse with me what you want to say so I can give you feedback on how it sounds . . ..'

HIGHLIGHTING THE PROBLEM-SOLUTION FOCUS

In reviewing their assessment and describing the CBT treatment model to the patient, the therapist will be implicitly emphasising the way in which therapy will be target-centred and quite actively focused on finding practical solutions to problems. While all other psychotherapies are in some sense problem-solution focused, in CBT this will be different from an approach such as person-centred counselling. In counselling the therapist traditionally provides a warm, empathic atmosphere to help the person explore problems, gain insight and then find the motivation to make the appropriate changes. Whereas the cognitive behaviour therapist must be skilled in counselling techniques, CBT will be slightly more prescriptive as it is assumed that (even with insight) the patient may need practical help or training to develop skills that promote change. For example, while counselling skills may help patients gain insight into the way a stressful lifestyle is taking its toll on their voice, it cannot be expected to make them aware of the many strategies that may be needed to reduce these stresses significantly. Lowering stress may require training in monitoring life activities, taking appropriate leisure, beginning regular exercise, using one or other form of muscular relaxation, applying rapid stress-control techniques, practising assertiveness in situations graded for level of difficulty and so on. Thus, at the start of treatment the therapist makes every effort to convey the therapeutic philosophy of deepening insight and self-knowledge in combination with practical strategies designed to solve specific problems and enhance change.

In recent times solution focused brief therapy has become a popular treatment model among speech and language therapists in the U.K. While this can be a useful approach that has much to offer in terms of a problem-solution emphasis, we feel it is often of limited use with many psychogenic voice disorder patients because it fails to comprehensively assess underlying or formative schemas as well as extensively employ the use of multiple cognitive behavioural treatment strategies.

EMPHASISING THE ROLE OF COLLABORATION AND SELF-HELP

In providing the client with a review of findings, through making the treatment model explicit and by highlighting the problem-solution focus, the therapist will implicitly emphasise the role of collaboration and self-help. It should be made clear to the client that CBT is not an approach like massage or reflexology or some other forms of speech and language therapy where the therapist *does* something that takes the problem away. It is, essentially, a collaborative venture. Therapist and patient work together, exploring problems, looking for solutions, agreeing on targets for change. Just as in the homework of voice exercises, the patient learns that in CBT some of the most important work of therapy goes on outside of individual sessions. In this process the client should become aware that the collaboration, target-setting and problem solving lead naturally to self-help. The approach helps therapists avoid falling into open-ended treatment contacts, boosts patient motivation and reduces the patient's natural tendency to become therapist dependent.

A particular benefit of this emphasis in therapy for the client is that it is very empowering. They can feel respected as someone capable of learning and changing. This can increase self-esteem and a sense of self-direction or self-control that can be an invaluable help in cases where anxiety and depression are related to feelings of low self-confidence and feelings of helplessness.

Finally, the emphasis can also add to the process of patient demystification. Patients should find answers to their questions and can test for themselves whether the cognitive behavioural view makes sense or produces results. In essence, the client should be made to feel 'an insider' in a process that deepens their self-understanding and creates positive change.

PROVIDING A TIME-LIMITED TREATMENT CONTRACT

With its problem-solution and target-centred orientation, CBT tends to be one of the briefer forms of therapy, and many practitioners find it valuable to make this clear from the outset. This clarifies what is being offered and should dispel any other expectations. Some therapists offer a specific number of sessions at the outset, for example, in Cognitive Analytic Therapy (Ryle 1990) the patient is offered a standard course of 16 sessions. Others offer an initial six sessions that are extended if, on review, it is believed that progress is being made. However, if this approach is used, the therapist should indicate at the outset something of the total number of sessions on offer. In this case it can be helpful to explain to the patient that results from CBT are usually achieved between 6–20 sessions and treatment normally concludes at this point.

Although some patients find it difficult to imagine that lifelong problems can be changed in such a short time, the majority appear to welcome the structure and focus this provides. For the majority, the brevity of treatment provides an incentive to make the most of the therapeutic meetings and to work hard at various self-help strategies between sessions.

Because the therapy is brief, transference problems are usually less of an issue than is the case in long-term psychotherapy, but when there are three or four sessions remaining in the contract, the patient will need reminding that the treatment is coming to a close. Raising the topic allows discussion of concerns the patient has about coping or continuing the progress without regular therapeutic contact. Although at the conclusion of treatment some patients will still feel the need for further support, the therapist will be able to emphasise that his or her role has been to help deepen their insight and to provide strategies for change and the rest is self-application and self-help which has to be done more and more independently of guidance from the therapist. The therapist can also offer a follow-up review in three months or suggest that he or she can be contacted and a further therapeutic contract arranged if there is either a crisis or if progress is not as good as expected. The review can be part of the voice review commonly used by speech and language therapists.

These suggestions are usually satisfactory for most patients and few abuse the arrangement or become unreasonably demanding of the therapist's time. However, when patients have not made satisfactory progress within the therapeutic contract, alternative therapies or referrals may have to be considered.

SUMMARY

This chapter describes a number of skills essential to CBT. It also offers guidelines that should be followed in order to perform competently as a cognitive behaviour therapist. Given their variety and complexity, the SLT will need to seek professional training and supervision to acquire these skills, which are listed below:

Check list of essential therapeutic skills and guidelines

- Creating a sound therapeutic relationship
- Thinking holistically and systematically and considering individual differences
- Using various forms of data collection, for example:

    Questionnaires
    Reflecting
    Listening
    Observing and questioning
    Questioning
    Socratic questioning and Socratic Dialogue
    Downward Arrow Techniques
    Constructive Questioning and Language
    Daily record sheets

- Formulating tentative hypotheses
- Providing a review of your thoughts, findings and formulations
- Making the treatment model explicit and highlighting the problem-solution focus
- Emphasising the role of collaboration and self-help
- Providing a time-limited treatment contract.

4 Assessment of Voice and Personal History

Having introduced the basic principles of CBT we will now put it more firmly into the context of the voice assessment. Typically the speech and language therapist's method of assessing the voice patient and reaching a diagnosis is arrived at by first having information from the otolaryngologist with regard to the condition and function of the larynx and then by taking a detailed case history. The otolaryngologist may have undertaken the laryngeal assessment alone or in collaboration with the speech and language therapist in the voice clinic. To complete the voice assessment the speech and language therapist may use a perceptual evaluation using a framework such as the Vocal Profile Analysis (Laver 1980) or the GRBAS measure (Hirano 1981), and may augment this with an acoustic analysis, through the use of instrumentation. Clearly there is a limited role for the latter in the aphonic patient, aside from demonstrating the potential for normal vocal-fold activity using vegetative behaviours such as coughs.

LARYNGEAL AND PERCEPTUAL PRESENTATION

The common physiological and perceptual features of psychogenic dysphonia and aphonia have been described in Tables 1.1 and 1.2, pages 2 and 3. Biofeedback in the form of a dynamic laryngoscopic view of the larynx may well be utilised by the speech and language therapist in the voice clinic as part of the assessment process. Vegetative phonatory behaviours may be used to explore the capabilities of the larynx as part of the diagnostic process and can be capitalised on further at the point of educating the patient about the dysphonia using video footage of the laryngeal assessment, (Rattenbury, Carding and Finn 2004). These vegetative behaviours will be detailed fully in Chapter 5 about symptomatic voice therapy.

VOICE CASE HISTORY

When taking a voice case history the speech and language therapist will want to ensure that information is elicited that relates to the presenting voice disorder, the medical history, as well as undertaking a perceptual assessment of voice. Most texts on the speech and language therapist's management of dysphonia include or refer to examples of case history forms (for example, Boone 1977; Colton & Casper 1996; Koschkee & Rammage 1997; Boone & McFarlane 2000; Martin & Lockhart 2000;

Mathieson 2001). These forms guide the therapist in taking information about the presenting voice disorder, medical and social history as well as suggesting areas of voice assessment. Although questions about environmental and emotional issues are considered to be important in the case history process, the detail and sophistication of the psychological interviewing recommended in voice texts is not always sufficient to reveal the causative factors. There is no text that guides the therapist towards a comprehensive psychosocial assessment for patients with voice disorders. The result is that therapy can be focused too often on the vocal symptoms, thus reinforcing the patients' view that this is a *mechanical* voice problem. The underlying causes perpetuating the dysphonia can too easily be neglected. Aronson, (1990b), eloquently reminds us of this

> . . . if we do not ask, and the patient does not volunteer the information, which they almost never do, then what other conclusion can we draw than that they have no psychologically related voice disorder? Our thinking becomes circular. If we do not ask about psychological problems, we do not hear about them. If we do not hear about them, we do not believe in them. And, if we do not believe in them; we do not ask about them.

(p. 288)

In this chapter we seek to redress the current lack of available psychological assessment tools for SLTs working with voice disorders by providing a framework that offers either a screening or full psychosocial assessment.

In brief, this chapter will extend the reader's understanding of the common aetiological features of a psychogenic voice disorder, (mentioned previously in Table 1.3, p. 4), and will provide the therapist with a psychosocial case history framework – for both screening or full assessment – that is sensitive to these aetiological features. The chapter also seeks to illustrate how the CBT assessment principles and therapist skills, explored more fully in the previous chapter, can be adopted by the SLT. With practice the SLT voice specialist can become increasingly adept at synthesising the CBT assessment tools and skills within the voice case history. In so doing the SLT will not only learn more about the predisposing, precipitating and perpetuating factors of the PVD, but will also enable the patient to appreciate these links. Thus, the therapist becomes better placed to then help the patient make the all-important cognitive and behavioural changes. Later chapters will explore some treatment modalities, again within a CBT approach, that can be applied to these patients with PVD.

A PSYCHOSOCIAL SCREENING TOOL AND FULL ASSESSMENT FOR VOICE DISORDERS

The position we take is that the standard voice case history should be extended to include more structured personal data collection, which we would consider to be a psychosocial screening, and that for some patients this is extended to allow for a full psychological history based on the cognitive behavioural model. The screening would involve a few well-structured questions, based on evidence of psychogenic voice disorder aetiological factors, which are sensitively and skilfully included in the standard voice case history.

The evidence from the common aetiological features of patients with psychogenic voice disorder is that they have wide ranging difficulties around their psychosocial functioning and, unless the therapist can question the patient with confidence in these areas, the diagnosis and subsequent therapy will be compromised. A full psychosocial interview takes time but often proves to be time well spent. If a therapist has opted to treat the voice symptomatically but finds after a few sessions that the voice therapy is not proving effective, it is probably because the therapist needs to know more about the aetiology and what is blocking remediation. If key questions have been asked at interview it is quite a logical step to reflect back on patients' responses, for example:

> *Before we continue with more voice exercises I would like to spend a little time reflecting on some of the things that may be going on in your life that could be contributing to the voice problem. I remember you said that you had felt very tired earlier in the year and that your job was becoming less enjoyable, so can we talk about this a little?*

If there had been no psychological questioning at the interview the therapist now has to focus attention on it for the first time. Arguably this is more disruptive to the flow of therapy.

What the therapist needs to find is a comfortable position where the voice case history is extended to allow for more sensitive and relevant data collection without straying completely into the field of clinical psychology. This has as much to do with time constraints as it has to do with professional appropriateness. For although we might advocate that a speech and language therapist, with guidance, practice and supervision, can become skilled in psychological interviewing there is not always the time in a busy clinic to be as comprehensive in the assessment areas as is required.

PSYCHOSOCIAL SCREENING

We advocate that some questions around psychosocial areas are included routinely in the voice case history. This allows the SLT to consider psychological factors that may have an influence on precipitating and perpetuating any voice disorder. The information gained from screening questions will enable the therapist to gauge whether fuller psychological assessment is necessary. Some screening questions should certainly be standard practice whenever a psychogenic voice disorder is suspected or when the therapist is making a differential diagnosis between a muscle tension dysphonia and a psychogenic voice disorder. However, since (as we say in Chapter 1) patients with muscle tension dysphonias will have some degree of stress in their lives, we would strongly recommend that psychosocial screening questions are included in the assessment of this patient group – regardless of whether the patient has secondary organic laryngeal changes. We would also recommend this screening assessment where the therapist felt that psychological factors might be perpetuating a primary organic voice disorder. There are, of course, patients whose voice disorders are clearly caused by structural or neurological impairment, such as papilloma or recurrent laryngeal nerve palsy, and there are patients who appear perfectly adjusted and relaxed. It can still be appropriate to include psychosocial questioning; in practice this part of the interview can be brief and the therapist's clinical judgement will gauge how much or how little probing is necessary. It may be that significant life stresses or personality traits do emerge and although these may not have been the causative factors of the dysphonia they could contribute to the maintenance of the voice disorder or impede the success of voice therapy if left unattended.

Psychosocial screening assessment recommended with the following:

- **psychogenic voice disorder suspected**
- **differential diagnosis between muscle tension dysphonia and PVD**
- **all muscle tension dysphonias**
- **brief questioning for primary organic based dysphonias**
- **all aphonics (but refer to Chapter 5 for the timing of the case history p. 95)**

FULL PSYCHOSOCIAL ASSESSMENT

In the majority of cases, sensitive, well-structured screening questions will offer valuable information that will be sufficient in enabling the SLT to manage the patient with regard to the predisposing, precipitating and perpetuating factors of their voice disorder. However, there will be patients with psychogenic voice disorders where, in order to appreciate the full aetiological factors and hence to offer true remediation, a fuller psychosocial assessment is required. The need for a full assessment may become apparent during the screening questions and in this case the therapist can direct the interview immediately to a more comprehensive psychosocial assessment. For other patients, despite the inclusion of screening questions at the initial case history, the full extent and complexity of the psychogenic nature of the voice disorder does not become apparent until therapy is underway. Perhaps the therapist begins to feel that there is more to the patient's story than has been told and this is blocking remediation. The areas needing closer examination may be the family background, early relationships or life events. In this instance the therapist may need to pause and redirect a session to a full psychosocial assessment. It is the minority of patients who will require this full level of psychosocial assessment and this chapter will include guidance on how and what information should be collected.

> **Full psychosocial assessment recommended when:**
>
> - It is clearly apparent from screening questions that there is a complex psychological history that needs to be explored in full, to identify the 3 Ps. This may be the case for either a psychogenic dysphonia or aphonia.
> - At a later stage when progress in therapy is not as anticipated from the initial screening.

THE ASSESSMENT OF PSYCHOSOCIAL AND COGNITIVE BEHAVIOURAL FEATURES

In terms of the personal history details there is now enough known from the literature to direct us in the areas in which we need to question the voice patient. In Table 1.3, we reported on a wide range of studies that have enabled us to recognise common aetiological features of the population who have psychogenic voice disorders. With this knowledge, the psychological voice assessment – both screening or full assessment can be more sensitively and appropriately focused. Thus, we will now elaborate on our understanding of these features and demonstrate how they can provide us with a more focused and comprehensive voice case history.

IDENTIFYING PREDISPOSING, PRECIPITATING AND PERPETUATING AETIOLOGICAL FEATURES OF PSYCHOGENIC VOICE DISORDERS

SIGNIFICANT LIFE EVENTS/STRESSES

Psychogenic voice disorders usually follow either an event of acute stress or are associated with stress over a long period of time (references, Table 1.3 p. 4). Typical major life events that we have seen have also involved isolation from a familiar environment and friends, usually the result of a house move, an unresolved family feud where the patient is prevented from or feels unable to resume a relationship with a family member or members, marital breakdown and bereavement. Role conflicts, promotion and new responsibilities at work are other common sources of stress. In particular, the stressful effect of loss, especially bereavement, is a most frequently occurring event and typically the patient is the daughter who is in some way still grieving for a parent. The bereavement may signify different things for the patient, such as the loss of a friend, comforter and confidante or remorse at not having been able to resolve anger or unfinished business. The bereavement has usually occurred in the recent past, perhaps within the last two years. Although this is the more common pattern, we have worked with cases where the bereavement has occurred up to 10 years before and in some cases during the patient's early life, maybe more than 20 years previously. In these cases the grieving may be incomplete or the effect of the death may have led to the formulation of negative schemas and distortions in thinking that have persisted into the present day and continue to colour the patient's behaviours and view of the world.

Assessment tips for SLT:

- **Probe for significant life changes that have occurred, particularly in the recent past, i.e. last two years.**
- **Look for tensions and conflicts with significant others that are unresolved and associated with inhibition, anger and difficulty expressing feelings/ views, etc. (See details in the following sections.)**
- **Questions should be specifically asked to identify bereavement(s).**

SYMPTOMS OF STRESS, ANXIETY AND PHYSICAL TENSION

As a consequence of the stressful life events, anxiety is an extremely common symptom, coupled with excessive muscular tension (see references, Table 1.3 p. 4). Hammarberg (1987) investigated musculoskeletal tension using pitch and quality characteristics of the voice and its possible origins and considered its impact on the possible alteration of voice production. Although the study focused on the adolescent male voice, the author concluded that the musculoskeletal tension that led to the altered voice production directly resulted from emotional conflict.

A study by Austin in 1997, which involved a structured interview with patients with a diagnosis of psychogenic voice disorder, gives useful illustrations of the laryngeal tension and tightness commonly felt by patients. Transcripts include the following examples from three patients who were describing what would happen to their throat and voice during situations that provoked anxiety for them:

'Voice disappears as it gets to the top of my mouth, it is a real strain to get it out.'
'I would have no voice, I would think first and then lose (my) voice because (my) throat tightens.'
'I can't imagine the words would come out, throat would go hard and tight.'

These quotes suggest an emotional physiological response that leads to the experience of the throat tightening with the consequence of dysphonia or loss of voice. There is a good deal already known about the relationship between increased muscle tension and the working of the larynx. A study of the mechanics of vocal fold tensioning in hyperfunctional dysphonia by Harris and Lieberman (1993) adds to our understanding of this link. This study explains how vocal fatigue and a loss of vocal range occur as the consequence of persistent patterns of vocal hyperfunction in stressed individuals. Furthermore, the study explains that these patterns of hyperfunction are frequently associated with postural problems, namely an extended head position and a kyphotic hump in the upper thoracic vertebrae, producing a cervicodorsal vertebral shelf.

Assessment tips for the SLT:

- **The therapist should question the patient about anxiety symptoms such as restlessness or agitation, panic attacks, breathlessness, headache, altered sleeping patterns, appetite and general feeling of wellbeing. N.B. A more comprehensive list of anxiety symptoms is included in Chapter 9, pages 157–8, in the description of anxiety disorders.**
- **An examination of posture and head and neck alignment, of the extrinsic laryngeal muscles and of breathing patterns is important to reveal the degree and location of inappropriate tension.**

FAMILY OR INTERPERSONAL RELATIONSHIP DIFFICULTIES

In our clinical sample (Butcher et al. 1987) we found that family and/or interpersonal relationship difficulties occurred very frequently and were usually the dominant feature in the history. Several patients had a poor marriage or experienced marital conflicts, their communication was poor and they shared very little with their partners. Others had a difficult or disturbed relationship with their child or children. In a few of these cases there was a disturbed mother/child relationship over issues of control. An outstanding feature was the immaturity of the child or children, most of whom were in their teens or early twenties. The parent usually had little independence, had a fragile identity and was highly controlled or dominated by the child. Andersson and Schalen (1998) also found that interpersonal conflicts related to family and work were important precipitating factors in psychogenic voice disorder.

Assessment tips for the SLT:

- **Examine close or important relationships.**
- **Look for any unresolved conflict or imbalance of power in relationships.**

DIFFICULTY EXPRESSING VIEWS OR EMOTIONS OR BEING ASSERTIVE AND SUPPRESSING ANGER AND FRUSTRATION

Many of the patients described above had difficulty in being assertive, expressing feelings of anger or resentment and personal views (see, for example, Butcher et al.

1987 where these were clearly demonstrated in at least eight of the 19 patients studied). This tendency often caused patients to have to passively accept an unfulfilling relationship without a means of protest. Aronson (1990a, p. 132) made a similar observation when he noted that a large number of patients showed 'difficulty in dealing maturely and openly with feelings of anger'. A study by House and Andrews (1988) more specifically details that the difficulty or event preceding the dysphonia commonly involves problems with self-expression or a 'conflict over speaking out'. They described this in the context of a specific stressful event where the patient has some strong commitment to the situation, such as a maintainer of family cohesion. When a conflict arises the patient is under pressure to speak out in order to continue that commitment but is inhibited through a fear of making matters worse. Their study of life events preceding psychogenic voice disorder showed that 54% of female patients reported experiencing a situation or difficulty involving a conflict over speaking out, while only 16% of a non-psychogenic voice disorder comparison group reported having a problem in this area of life.

In one study, Austin's (1997) group of psychogenic voice patients were given scenarios that would involve speaking out. They were asked to describe what emotions they would experience in these different social situations and how their voice production would be affected. Their responses illustrate a fear of the emotions and the consequences associated with speaking out and also a fear that the voice would let them down. For example, 'I don't think I can say that, don't like upsetting anyone. Inside me I think I should do it, but feel very uncomfortable. I don't want my friend hurt. My voice would be really, really tight.'

Furthermore, Austin found that one of the most striking features about this group of patients was their fear of the expression of negative emotions, such as anger, and their fears of rejection, such as losing friends as a consequence of speaking out, and their inability to deal with these emotions. For example:

'If I did speak out I would squash the person, get very angry, so it's best to keep calm and not say anything.'
'I would be worried about hurting their feelings and losing their friendship.'
'I want to please people and not wanting to disappoint.'

Austin's patients tended to use avoidance as the mechanism to refrain from speaking out, for example:

'It would be best to say nothing.'
'I don't think I can say that, inside me I think I should do it but feel very uncomfortable, so leave it to my wife.'

In highlighting so clearly the feature of conflict over speaking out, the study also adds support to the view that those individuals whose predisposition or social learning make it difficult for them to express views or feelings may be more likely to experience voice disorders than the general population.

Assessment tips for the SLT:

- Explore whether the patients tend to share problems and anxieties or whether they tend to keep them to themselves. How good are the patients at saying how they feel and giving their opinion?
- Are the patients experiencing 'a conflict over speaking out' and therefore keeping quiet when in fact they would like to express their feelings?
- Be observant to signs of suppressed anger or frustration.

POWERLESSNESS AND HELPLESSNESS

The difficulty that these patients have in expressing their feelings probably contributes to feelings of powerlessness and helplessness, (Butcher et al. 1993). This may be particularly important psychologically, as it is now widely accepted that feelings of powerlessness and helplessness or the loss of freedom to act are associated with emotional disturbance and conditions of anxiety and depression, (Rotter 1966; Seligman 1975; Yalom 1980; Bandura 1989).

Austin's (1997) transcripts also illustrate these patients' disbelief in their own self-worth, which contributes to their feelings of helplessness and powerlessness:

'Why would people listen to my conversation?'
'I often feel part of the problem and would like to be part of the answer.'
'I never think I am good enough and could always do better.'

Importantly, Austin's (1997) study has suggested that many conflicts, like those associated with conflict over speaking out and helplessness experienced by her patients, arose from **background influences** or social conditioning. She gives several illuminating examples including:

'It's to do with upbringing, we weren't taught to stand up and speak out even at school. . .(women) were supposed to be seen and not heard.'
'It's not the done thing, British reserve, upbringing, era and age group.'
'My father used to raise his voice and it was terrifying, I can't remember the last time I raised mine.'
'My father was head of the family and me and mum had to march behind him. I was made to feel very important as long as I was behind him.'

Assessment tips for the SLT:

- How good are the patients at asking for their needs to be met?
- Does the patient present with low self-esteem or feel undervalued?

THE BURDEN OF RESPONSIBILITY

We have found (Butcher & Elias 1983; Butcher et al. 1987) that many patients have taken the onus of responsibility in their family or marriage, but staggered under the burden. In some cases, they felt that they were married to passive or uncooperative partners who took little or no responsibility for the home or for such things as disciplining the children. Another common and related feature to emerge from our observation of this population is where the patient is caught in a stressful relationship with an elderly, dependent mother or father. The patients had been left with, or had taken on, the main responsibility for looking after their parent. They tended to have little or no support in doing this and, even when support was available, they felt they had to take the main responsibility for care. This sense of responsibility can also extend beyond the family. A telling quote from one patient in Austin's (1997) study was that 'I don't refuse friends favours, I would do it at any cost. If I had to refuse, I wouldn't have a voice because I would lose it because my throat tightens.'

OVER-COMMITMENT AND HELPLESSNESS

We have also noted when assessing the female dysphonics in our study that these women not only tend to take on the main burden of responsibility within the family, but are also often unable to make changes in an unsatisfactory situation owing to their lack of assertiveness. A similar impression was formed by House and Andrews (1988) who noted that, 'these women have a tendency to become involved in a social network in which they were over-committed, but relatively powerless' (p.317). Although House and Andrews did not postulate what early experience may have led to 'this over-devoted style in relationships', a comment from one of Austin's patients may suggest a possible answer. 'From childhood I was taught if people need help you should always help. If people don't help they are. . .(an) arsehole.'

We have frequently noted cases where the woman is juggling a job, often when working in a stressful environment or long hours, as well as having to be a housewife and mother. For many of these patients their loss of voice increased the stresses at work because they were no longer able to perform their duties adequately.

Assessment tips for the SLT:

- **The therapist needs to hear about the patient's lifestyle and responsibilities and how well the patient is balancing and coping with these.**
- **Are these elements of their life enjoyable or have they become a burden? Are there specific stressful responsibilities and what support is the patient really getting from others?**
- **Does the patient invite support or tend to shoulder the responsibilities alone? Does the patient feel well supported in close relationships?**

TRANSITION INTO ADULTHOOD

It has also been our unreported clinical observations that there may be a specific population of teenagers who experience voice disorder or voice loss and where it is often difficult, even with hindsight, to identify a cause. Typically these are young people in their late teens and sometimes early twenties who arrive in the clinic with a voice disorder or aphonia of sudden onset. In our experience these cases have usually been young girls, but we have met a smaller number of boys in this age range with similar presentations. We have sometimes noted environmental and emotional factors associated with these cases although these certainly do not operate in all cases. These young people are living at home and in some instances are beginning their first job or their first sexual relationship. There is often caring and concerned support from the parents. The patient may be demonstrating some signs of anxiety. Although compliant in voice therapy the patient may present rather shyly, seeming rather young and naïve, and be unwilling or unable to communicate freely. In virtually all cases the voice has returned, sometimes slowly, through a firm, reassuring, empathetic and confident approach by the therapist usually focusing on freeing the vocal tract and the voice. However, the therapist has been none the wiser afterwards as to the underlying triggers for the voice loss apart from hypothesising that it has a link with some difficulty in the transition from childhood into adulthood and inhibitions around the expression of feelings. There is some support for these clinical observations in a study by Kinzl et al. (1988). These authors found that in their group of 'hysterical patients' a majority reported stress situations that were 'most commonly caused by events related to maturation processes, such as leaving home, vocational career etc.' (p. 34).

Assessment tips for the SLT:

- **Find out if the young person has recently left home, begun employment or further education, has started a relationship and whether this is a first relationship. Are there any signs of anxiety around any of these areas?**
- **Does the young person have close friendships; are there any confidants (parent/grandparent/aunt/friend)?**
- **Ask questions about the young person's personality; shy/nervous/confident/talkative.**
- **What kind of relationship does he or she have with their parents and siblings?**

THE EFFECT OF THE DYSPHONIA

It is acknowledged that the voice disorder can be a distressing experience and that in itself this experience exacerbates the condition as Aronson (1990a) explains: 'the patient's frustration and anger elevate musculoskeletal tension, and whatever primary organic or psychogenic voice disorder existed up to that point is worsened to an even greater degree of severity' (p.140). In Chapter 1 (page 3) we explained how lowered mood or mild–moderate depression can occur as a consequence of the voice disorder and that the voice disturbance may prevent the patient from working normally as well as reduce their social integration.

Table 4.1: Summary of common aetiological features of psychogenic voice disorders and the implications for assessment

Common Aetiological Features	Considerations for Assessment
1. Significant life stresses/events	• There may be one or several major life events. Look for life changes, especially in the recent past, for example, family feuds, isolation from friends or bereavement.
2. Symptoms of stress over a period of time leading to anxiety and physical tension.	• Anxiety symptoms, e.g. panic attacks, breathlessness, headaches, changes in sleep patterns and appetite, distractibility, dizziness, palpitations, globus pharyngeus. Fatigue and changes in general health, diet and presence of gastro-oesophageal reflux. • Examination of posture, extrinsic laryngeal muscles and breathing patterns.
3. Family or interpersonal relationship difficulties.	• Examine close or important relationships; look for any unresolved conflict or imbalance of power.
4. Difficulty in expressing views and emotions and in being assertive. Suppressing anger and frustration.	• Does the patient express wants and feelings? Does the patient share troubles? Are there things that the patient has left unsaid particularly where the patient feels angry or frustrated? Is there 'a conflict over speaking out' with a significant other?
5. Burden of responsibility. Overcommitment and helplessness.	• Learn about the patient's lifestyle and responsibilities. How well does the patient balance and cope with different responsibilities? Is the patient caring for someone or for several people? What help is the patient getting? Are they stuck in one approach to things? Does the patient invite support or not? Does the patient balance needs, relaxation and leisure time? Does the patient have low self-esteem or feel undervalued?
6. The effect of the dysphonia	• What does the voice disorder mean for the patient? Is it causing additional stress and how is the patient coping with it? Has it led to changes in the patient's work, lifestyle or social network?

Remember this is a guide and not a comprehensive list. Be ready to listen for additional clues.

Assessment tips for the SLT:

- Explore how the patient is coping with the voice disorder and how he or she views it.
- Find out whether any external changes have occurred as a *result* of the voice disorder, for example having to make changes in their job or an avoidance of socialising with friends.
- Does the patient feel more isolated as a result of the voice disorder?

PSYCHOSOCIAL HISTORY TAKING WITHIN A VOICE CASE HISTORY FRAMEWORK

THERAPIST SKILLS

By taking into account the predisposing, precipitating and perpetuating factors of psychogenic voice disorders, described above, it is possible to offer the SLT a more sensitive, psychologically oriented case history form. However, before exploring this orientation, several things should be borne in mind. Above all, what follows must be considered against a backdrop of sound counselling skills. Many thoughts and feelings that patients bring to therapy are only half formulated and understood, are difficult to express and are often being described for the first time. The therapist will need to listen for clues in what patients are trying to describe and also to have a sensitive ear and keen eye for underlying themes or hidden messages. The skillful interviewer must be able to listen, observe and formulate hypotheses for testing. Thus, it is less helpful to think of a prescriptive set of questions that the speech and language therapist should ask. Instead it is important to be responsive to the patient, listening to what is being said, speculating about what the patient may be alluding to, watching for changes in speech, posture or affect and then weaving in pertinent questions to clarify a point or draw out information.

The patient will, to some extent, influence the structure of the interview. For example, if the patient is particularly distressed about a certain issue in his or her life the therapist may need to acknowledge this and then sensitively redirect the patient to other areas of questioning, in order to build a comprehensive picture. Thus, although we can suggest areas in which to examine, and indeed perhaps some questions to ask, the way in which the therapist introduces different areas of questioning and the approach taken with each patient must be appropriately gauged through active listening. Therefore, the initial interview takes the form of information seeking and the speech and language therapist employs good counselling skills while gathering and processing a wide range of information. The therapist's skills necessary for undertaking a CBT style interview were explored in Chapter 3. Essentially though, the speech and language therapist will be skilled in:

- creating a sound therapeutic relationship
- thinking holistically and systematically about psychological processes, with consideration of the 3 Ps (the predisposing, the precipitating and the perpetuating factors)
- reflection, in order to encourage, to clarify and to begin to invite insight
- attentive listening and observing. This enables the therapist to be alert to hidden messages or meanings, make intuitive connections and then explore these further through focused questions.
- good questioning; using both open and closed questions and knowing when and how to pose a sensitive question. The therapist may also learn to be skilled in Socratic questions, downward arrow technique and the use of constructive questions (Chapter 3, pp. 46–8). The CBT model requires comprehensive questioning covering *cognitive, emotional and behavioural features.*
- using daily record sheets
- formulating tentative hypotheses.

Many of these skills will already be embedded in the practice of the SLT working with voice, but some will need to be acquired and developed through access to training and/ or supervision from a CBT practitioner. Although we are recommending that psychosocial history taking should be included in the initial assessment, it is a feature of CBT that further questioning, reflection and data collection will be central to much of the subsequent treatment. This concept is familiar to the speech and language therapist who finds that increasing personal data is elicited once a rapport has been established during treatment sessions.

SCREENING ASSESSMENT VERSUS FULL PSYCHOSOCIAL ASSESSMENT

Since it is our view that speech and language therapists will benefit from asking most patients with voice disorders for a degree of psychosocial information, we advocate that some screening questions or prompts could be incorporated into most voice case histories. The standard voice case history proforma in Table 4.4 includes sample screening prompts that may provide some valuable psychological history and help the therapist towards a tentative hypothesis about aetiology and a more complete therapy plan. This process of weaving a few well-focused questions into the voice case history is likely to be sufficient for the majority of patients.

A full psychosocial assessment is reserved for those patients requiring a more detailed psychological understanding. As stated earlier in this chapter, the need for this will either become apparent as the SLT elicits answers to the screening questions or will be indicated later during therapy.

STRUCTURING THE INTERVIEW

There is usually a logical structure to formulating the case history although the experienced SLT becomes increasingly able to work flexibly within this structure

Table 4.2: A standard voice case history with a psychosocial framework

With psychosocial screening prompts pp. 73–8

Presenting voice disorder

Onset and history of voice problem, including any history of previous voice disturbance
Description of present problem, variation of problem, triggers, etc.
Description of voice use. Hobbies, sports and interests

Related health issues

Medical information
Suggestions of anxiety symptoms
General health, including depression or lowered mood

Voice assessment

Including observation of breathing, posture and tension sites as well as assessment of voice
Assessment/palpation of laryngeal muscles to detect musculoskeletal tension

Family background

- brief family tree
- key relationships/significant figures

Personal history

- events around time of onset of voice disorder
- significant life stresses, e.g. bereavement, changes in job or at home, changes in responsibilities
- important relationships, including relationships where there may be a difficulty voicing feelings, unresolved conflicts or imbalance of power. Evidence of 'conflict over speaking out'
- juggling responsibilities or carrying a burden of responsibility including ability to set limits or invite support

according to the patients' responses. In Table 4.2 and Table 4.3 we provide examples of a framework for a voice case history that takes into account the psychosocial areas relevant in voice disorders from the evidence base that we described earlier in the aetiological studies. The framework described in Table 4.2 incorporates familiar areas of a standard voice case history, within which we would advocate the inclusion of psychosocial screening questions. This is further extended to allow for a full psychosocial assessment, described in Table 4.3 and Table 4.4.

Whether the therapist is conducting a screening or a full psychosocial assessment, it will be necessary at some point in the interview to probe for clues to stressful events preceding the onset of the dysphonia. However, it is probably best to begin by orientating the interview towards the medical history and direct voice information since the patient will be anticipating that line of questioning and it is a neutral area. The psychological questioning will then follow more comfortably when a rapport has been established. The speech and language therapist has obtained the history of the voice problem and can then gently turn the questioning to more personal probing. If patients

Table 4.3: A voice case history extended for full psychosocial assessment

Standard (with psychosocial prompts)	**Presenting voice disorder** Onset and history of voice problem, including any history of previous voice disturbance Description of present problem, variation of problem, triggers, etc. Description of voice use. Hobbies, sports and interests
	Related health issues Medical information Suggestions of anxiety symptoms General health, including depression or lowered mood
	Voice assessment Including observation of breathing, posture and tension sites as well as assessment of voice Assessment/palpation of laryngeal muscles to detect musculoskeletal tension
Extended	**Family background** • relationship with mother and father, type of person, current contact, etc. • family tree, number of siblings, type of relationship(s), current contact, etc. • general home environment • other significant figures, (e.g. grandparents, aunts, foster parents, carers) • family life events, (e.g. separation/divorce of parents, death of siblings/parents, relocation)
	Personal history • early development, family, cultural background and social relationships • personality as a child (e.g. shy/outgoing, confident/nervous, etc.) • transition to adulthood; identify changes, leaving home, etc. • personality prior to symptom onset (e.g. assertiveness/ability to express views and emotions/tendency to suppress anger and frustration) • events around time of onset of voice disorder • significant life stresses, e.g. bereavement, changes in job or at home, changes in responsibilities • marriage(s) and children • important relationships, including relationships where they may be a difficulty voicing feelings, unresolved conflicts or imbalance of power; evidence of 'conflict over speaking out' • current social circumstances • employment history • use of leisure time, ability to relax or pace oneself • juggling responsibilities or carrying a burden of responsibility including ability to set limits or invite support • self-esteem and feelings of self-worth

offer comments such as 'it's worse when I'm all stressed up' or 'it all started when there was a row at work', the speech and language therapist can store this away and then reflect it back when beginning to ask for personal data. The experienced therapist will not be rigid in the case history taking. Although there is some value in systematic questioning, a single question may elicit information at multiple levels. If the therapist is actively listening, it is possible to draw out parts of the personal history during, for example, a discussion around the voice history.

Psychosocial assessment areas

What now follows are areas commonly included in a voice case history but with guidance and examples as to how these areas may be extended for a more comprehensive psychosocial assessment. This guidance covers more of the extended case history areas that are listed in Table 4.3, and therefore the full detail of all that follows will be needed for only a minority of voice patients. Nevertheless, a familiarity with this information will be useful to SLTs with all their voice assessments, and some of what follows includes examples of the screening questions that are in the Standard voice case history proforma in Table 4.4.

PRESENTING VOICE DISORDER, DESCRIPTION OF PRESENT PROBLEM AND VARIATION IN PROBLEM

These areas are commonly included in a voice case history. As patients tend to recall the immediate voice problem it is important to ask the patient to think back as carefully as possible to the time when they began to notice voice problems. It is also important to ask whether they had ever had voice difficulties during previous occasions. Sometimes patients will be rather dismissive about this, 'Oh, my voice has never been good', so the speech and language therapist must ask the patient to be more specific about what that means, how the voice has varied and if there has been a pattern, what does the patient mean by 'not good' and when did the patient first notice a voice change. Through building a thorough picture of any previous periods of voice disturbance or voice loss the therapist will be collecting important information that may contribute to the diagnosis of a psychogenic voice disorder. The therapist will need to explore the circumstances of these spells of voice disturbance. Previous bouts of dysphonia and aphonia, in the absence of a throat infection and particularly when identified as being connected to periods of stress, will be an important diagnostic cue.

DESCRIPTION OF VOCAL USE – INCLUDING WORK, HOBBIES, SPORTS AND SINGING

When collecting this type of information the therapist will be on the look out for clues about the patient's lifestyle. Is this patient limited to social contact with their spouse? Is the patient balancing different roles in their life: work, mother, housewife? If the patient discloses limited information, 'No, I don't have to use my voice at work a great deal, just on the telephone', probe for more.

'And what about after work, who is at home? Are you a chatty person with your friends? What do you do in your leisure time?'

The therapist is building up a picture not only of voice use and potential areas of vocal misuse, but also piecing together the patient's social network and lifestyle. The need for the therapist to be attentive is illustrated in the example of a 30-year-old man with vocal fatigue. He described his demanding career and presented himself as a driven or 'Type A' personality, preferring to be busy, disliking slack times at work and living life in the fast lane. When recounting his social life he listed a lot of sport and the therapist could have been forgiven for assuming he was achieving a healthy balance of work and relaxation. Yet a little more questioning revealed that the sport was all active and aggressive, squash, aerobics and weight training where the tendency might be to increase laryngeal tension. Even when he included golf on his list he mentioned 'my game isn't very good when I'm all tensed up', suggesting that this sport did not necessarily relax him. In this interview this information was reflected back when the therapist was explaining the connection between muscle tension and dysphonia and encouraged the patient to see that equating relaxation with sport can be misleading.

HEALTH AND MEDICAL INFORMATION – INCLUDING ANXIETY SYMPTOMS, GENERAL HEALTH AND LOWERED MOOD

These areas should not be underestimated in their value for expanding on the psychological aspects that may be underpinning the voice disorder. In addition to the more obvious questioning regarding any upper respiratory tract infections, smoking, drinking and serious illness, the therapist should look at areas where there is often a relationship with stress. Clearly the SLT must be observant of symptoms that may have an organic cause, but assuming that the therapist is mindful of these links and follows appropriate lines of questioning or medical investigation, the following is a list of areas that may give useful clues about reactions to stress with suggested questions:

Sleep pattern	*'What is your sleeping like?'*
	'Has it changed?'
Appetite/diet	*'How is your appetite?'*
	'Do you have regular meal breaks/do you miss meals or eat on the run?'
Headache/Migraine	*'Do you get many headaches or migraine? How often would you say that was?'*
	'What do you think triggers these?'
Breathlessness	*'Do you ever get out of breath, during exercise or at other times?'*
Panic attacks	*'Do you ever get panicky feelings or perhaps feelings of butterflies in your tummy, feeling hot and sweaty or palpitations or feeling faint?'*
Tendency to worry	*'Do you think you are a worrier?'*
General wellbeing	*'How do you feel in general?'*
	'How are your energy levels?'
	'Have you been feeling low or tearful?'

The therapist should be confident in direct questioning. Once patients have settled into the interview they will usually respond well to this.

THE VOICE ASSESSMENT – INCLUDING BREATH, POSTURE AND VOCAL TRACT TENSION

Returning to the voice, therapists will use their preferred choice of perceptual voice assessment. Observation and assessment of posture will be included and it is appropriate to ask about pain or tension in the neck, shoulder and back as well as tension or clenching in the jaw. Although of direct relevance to musculoskeletal tension affecting the free vocal tract, this information is also touching again on stress symptoms. Similarly, information about posture at work, slouching over a desk, straining for the telephone, a lot of driving, may reveal more about lifestyle, personality and anxiety symptoms as well as about muscle posture and tension.

If an infant school teacher is telling you that she is getting to the end of each school day with a headache, tense neck and shoulders and vocal fatigue, she is probably telling you that her body is not free from tension and that there may be poor postural habits. She may also be telling you that her energy levels are low and that she may be finding it difficult to control the class. This information may have told you that this lady is tired, with several stress symptoms and is balancing various demands of family and work. Either at this point, or during the next section of the interview, the therapist would do well to enquire directly,

> *'How are you finding the class.' 'What do you feel about your job at the moment?' 'Do you enjoy it?'*

It is also necessary to look beyond the muscle tension experienced in the classroom and look to what is happening in her life that may be contributing to this state.

If the speech and language therapist has been trained in laryngeal palpation, a physical examination of the extrinsic laryngeal muscles is likely to be built into the voice assessment. The therapist will locate areas of muscle tension as well as acknowledging discomfort as muscle groups are palpated. Since, generally speaking, patients are more willing to accept a connection between muscle tension and a voice disorder, than stress or emotional factors, it can be helpful if the therapist uses the physical examination and palpation in order to discuss the tension in the laryngeal muscles. This can offer the therapist an opportunity for enquiring about stressful life events (see pp. 61 and 77), that may have contributed to the increased muscle tension and thus the voice disorder.

PERSONAL HISTORY

In preparing to take personal information the therapist will need first to gain the patient's cooperation and some trust. The therapist will probably need to give some explanation before shifting the focus of the interview to personal details. It is seldom necessary at this point to indulge the patient in lengthy academic connections between the dysphonia and stress, which may incline the patient to be guarded or defensive. The therapist will gauge the extent and manner of the explanation that is given to the patient. For example, a responsive and stressed patient may be only too pleased to be given the opportunity to get things off their chest and will only need a little prompting:

'Let's just look at a few things in your life at the moment'

or

'I would like to ask a little more about yourself and then I'll explain what I think may be the problem with your voice.'

If the patient is more guarded or is expressing the opinion that the dysphonia is a mechanical problem, the therapist may need to coax the patient, for example:

'We know that voices can be affected by too much muscle tension so it's a good idea to look at anything in your life that may be contributing to tension.'

or

'In a few minutes I'm going to try to explain what I think the problem is with your voice, but first I think it's important to ask you a little more about yourself.'

If the focus is deliberately manoeuvred to the physical manifestation, muscle tension, the patient is often more accepting of the interview.

There are some patients who will have divulged personal information earlier in the interview, almost as soon as they sit down and with little prompting. Therefore, the therapist can easily return to some of this information, for example:

'You mentioned earlier that you tend to get worked up over things, and I wondered if we could just look at what kind of things upset you.' 'You told me just now that your father died last year, and I wanted to ask you how you are coping with that.'

Since the therapist will want to have a degree of flexibility in the case history taking, in order to be appropriately responsive, the detailed personal data may have been collected as the issue arose at an earlier part of the interview. In the case of the patient who clearly wants to talk about an area of concern and this is interfering with effective data collection, the therapist may acknowledge this and defer them to this part of the interview, for example:

'Yes, I think your feelings towards your husband may be relevant but I wonder if I could just ask you a little more about your voice and then we could talk about these feelings some more.'

SIGNIFICANT LIFE STRESSES – EVENTS PRECEDING THE VOICE PROBLEM

Relationship Difficulties; Difficulties Expressing Views and Voicing Opinion

Questions around these areas are key to learning about possible causative factors. Direct, broad questioning is useful initially, for example:

> '*I wonder if you could tell me whether there have been any significant changes in your life over the past couple of years or so? Have you had any bereavements, have there been any changes in your job or at home?*'

As information is forthcoming the therapist can continue with appropriate questioning. This may be the first time that the patient considers a relevant connection between the voice disorder and events that have occurred some time before.

Questions also need to be focused towards events that more immediately preceded the dysphonia. Aronson (1990b) offers his advice with questions that he has found to be useful:

> '*Think back to when your voice trouble started. What was going on at that time that might have upset you?*'
> '*Is there anyone at home or at work whom you have been having problems with, such as your partner, children, parents, in-laws, colleagues, or supervisors? Have you had trouble expressing your feelings to these people? Have you been concerned about your health or the health of your family, or career, or your finances?*'

(p. 289)

There will be some instances when the voice therapist needs to take an extensive family and personal history, including all the areas suggested in Table 4.3. However, it is more often sufficient in the interview to obtain a broad family tree including sufficient social and personal detail in order to reveal potential key areas where there could be unresolved difficulties, past or present, so that the therapist can begin to hypothesise as to the background, cause and maintenance of the voice disorder. In the knowledge that our early life experiences shape our cognitive, emotional and behavioural responses to present day situations, it will sometimes be necessary to explore more of the family background and personal history (Table 4.3) in subsequent sessions. Perhaps this is the case where the patient is experiencing relationship difficulties or where the therapist detects a conflict over speaking out. The therapist will be looking to see what earlier experiences or personality traits may have influenced the current event. In addition to the questions suggested by Aronson, we would add the following:

> '*Are your parents alive?*'
> '*Do you have brothers and sisters?*'
> '*How would you describe your father (mother, brother, sister, wife)?*'
> '*What sort of person is he/she?*'
> '*How do you get on?*'

'Has your relationship with your (father, mother, daughter, etc.) changed in recent years?'
'How good are you at telling people what you want or how you feel?'
'Are there some situations where you find it more difficult to express your feelings?'
'Are there some people in your life to whom you find it difficult to speak your mind?'

Burden of Responsibility, Over-commitment and Helplessness

During the interview it may become apparent that the patient is tending to shoulder the burden of responsibility within the family, with friends or at work. Sometimes when discussing the significant life events in the preceding couple of years or the current stressors in the patient's life it can be seen that the patient is tending to take on a substantial caring role to others, perhaps at their own expense. If this is the picture that is emerging the therapist may wish to reflect this back sympathetically and then extend the questioning in this area, for example:

'It sounds as if you are good at looking after other people's needs. . .It sounds as if people tend to rely on you to give them support. Where do you get your support from?'
or
'Who would you turn to for your support?'

If the therapist is detecting a tendency towards over-commitment to others and perhaps the patient is also describing some physical and emotional fatigue, it may be useful to question a little more in the area of assertiveness. For example:

'How good are you at asking for support for yourself?'
'Are you able to say "no" when people ask for your help? How does saying "no" make you feel?'
'What time do you have for yourself? Are there any things that you do for yourself that make you feel good?'

PATIENT'S OWN OPINION

Sometimes the patient has a good idea about the cause of the voice problem, but in all of the rounds of visits to the GP and ENT department he has not been given the opportunity to suggest it. Asking the patient directly is often quite revealing:

'What do you think may be causing the voice problem?'
or
'Have you got any theories or ideas about what might be causing your voice problem?'

Quite often, and early in the voice case history, patients will volunteer that they feel the problem is to do with stress. In this case the therapist may invite the patients to expand on their view or may like to acknowledge it and defer more discussion until an appropriate time in the interview, by saying, for instance, *'Well, you could be right. May I come back to that point in a few minutes.'* Asking what the patients feel is wrong with their voice can also reveal fears that they have throat cancer, etc., and provides the therapist with an opportunity of offering both reassurance and alternative cognitive behavioural interpretations of voice loss.

SUBSEQUENT DATA COLLECTION AND QUESTIONNAIRES

In our explanation of CBT we have already said that as well as relying on good interviewing and history taking skills the therapist should be skilled in collecting data through standard questionnaires and the use of daily record sheets. As well as building up a picture of when and how the voice disorder may have originated, the therapist also needs to know how the originating problem may have influenced the thoughts, emotions and behavioural responses of the patient. Although the well focused questions, described in this chapter, will go a long way to collecting this information, the therapist will find that questionnaires and daily record sheets can be a useful adjunct. These are unlikely to be given to the patient during the initial case history but can be used in subsequent sessions when the therapist has embarked on a therapeutic course. We have already mentioned several questionnaires, including the HADS, all of which can be quickly administered by the speech and language therapist. In Chapters 6, 7 and 8 we give examples of how both questionnaires and record sheets can be used in assessing and treating anxiety and lowered mood associated with voice disorder.

Finally, it is worth saying here, that the speech and language therapist may occasionally identify a patient during assessment who appears to have a more complex psychopathology. We have therefore devoted Chapter 9 to look in some detail at different psychological disorders with the specific intention of helping the speech and language therapist decide when it is and is not appropriate to treat certain patients.

CONCLUDING THE INTERVIEW

IS THERE MORE TO ADD?

The way in which the initial interview is ended is an important consideration. If the psychosocial questioning has led to a lot of discussion, the therapist may like to ask whether the patient feels there is anything important that has not been covered. If, throughout the interview, the therapist has appeared to be genuinely concerned, empathic and understanding, the patient may now feel ready to go into issues which would have been difficult to discuss at the outset.

THANKING THE PATIENT

Whether conducting a screening or a full psychosocial assessment, on occasions it will be obvious that the patient has found the interview emotionally demanding. This may be the first time that the patient has confided to anyone. Perhaps the patient has described events which he or she would rather forget or has been tearful and may regret showing emotion in front of a stranger. In these situations the therapist should find a way of showing that he or she recognises how demanding the interview has been. It is important not to leave the patient feeling vulnerable or exposed. The therapist may stress the confidentiality of the session and may also choose to thank the patient for sharing his or her thoughts and for being prepared to be open even though it may have felt uncomfortable. Alternatively, the therapist may apologise for having to ask questions which were clearly upsetting, acknowledging this by saying,

> *'I'm sorry I've had to ask you so many questions. I can understand that this interview has not been easy.'*

Simple feedback of this sort can be reassuring to the patient and can help him or her feel that it has been worthwhile. This will be particularly so if the therapist explains that it has helped to formulate ideas about the cause of the problem and how it can be treated.

REFLECTING, EXPLAINING AND PROVIDING A TENTATIVE FORMULATION

Whatever the demands of the interview have been, the patient will be expecting some answers to the problem and will be looking for reassurance. The therapist should make every effort to meet these needs. A good way to start is by explaining voice production to the patient and it may be useful to emphasise the role of the muscles and their sensitivity to increased body tension. In relating the picture back to the patient it is important to explain the clinical diagnosis of the larynx and to explain that the patient does not have cancer.

One of the best ways to then explain things to the patient is to give a brief summary of what has been covered in the session, selecting what appear to be the important explanatory or causal factors in the voice disorder and suggesting that while future meetings will probably add more detail to the picture, it is possible at this stage to offer a tentative interpretation or formulation. If, throughout the interview the therapist has been conscious of thinking in terms of the overarching holistic model and has been asking questions around life events, interpersonal relationships, cognitions, emotions, physical symptoms and behavioural reactions, he or she will usually find that it is not too difficult to make the right connections and to offer a formulation based on the gathered information. The formulation should be given in simple terms with appropriate illustrations to help the patient understand what is being said. For instance, the therapist can illustrate the link between muscular tension and dysphonia by demonstrating vocal strain.

In presenting a psychological interpretation, it is important to reassure the patient that the therapist is not suggesting that the problem is 'all in the mind' or that the patient is mentally unbalanced. This would be an unreasonable conclusion and a patient left with that view is unlikely to be a willing partner in therapy. Again this issue is best dealt with when the formulation is summarised and by giving clear examples. One way of doing this is by highlighting the fact that, while people usually cope well with a reasonable amount of short periods of stress, they are often adversely affected emotionally and physically when stresses become multiple, protracted or intense. Just as physical conditions like a headache or upset stomach can be caused by worry and stress, so can a voice disorder, since the voice is particularly sensitive to emotion. The therapist can explain that a psychological assessment and view of the voice disorder is concerned with understanding in some depth the life stresses, worries and emotions that might be causing the voice problem and with finding practical strategies to reduce these stresses. It is best not to be too dogmatic when offering a hypothesis, rather to present views as a possibility for the patient to consider and thus encouraging their self-reflection. The therapist should conclude by checking with the patient how plausible this summing up has been. In Chapter 3 we suggested saying something at this point like:

'I don't know if this way of looking at things makes sense to you? Have I missed anything that feels important?'

In helping the patient make the connection between psychological wellbeing and voice, Aronson also recognises the importance we should place on this part of the interview. In his words we should, 'educate patients about the relationship between throat muscle tension and psychologic stress, assure them that we do not think they are mentally unbalanced, and reassure them that the voice disorder is not their fault' (1990b, p. 289). Whether or not the speech and language therapist intends to manage the psychological therapy with supervision or to refer the patient directly to psychology, we would agree with Aronson that speech and language therapists 'have a responsibility for being the "advanced party", for breaking new ground, and for helping the patient to discover, perhaps for the first time, that further help is needed' (1990a, p. 324). It is essential that the SLT does not default from explaining the working hypothesis, i.e. the belief that psychological factors are strongly influencing the patient's voice disorder through their influence on physiological functioning.

We said in the previous chapter that helping patients make more sense of their problems not only helps to demystify the patient's complaint and to therefore reduce uncertainty and stress, but it also enables them to make sense, and best use of the CBT approach. This summing up after the assessment is therefore an essential part of the therapy process and if done well, with a reflective patient, can go a great way towards a positive outcome. The case history of Sue, described briefly in Chapter 5 and fully in Chapter 10, pp. 191–4, is an example of a successful CBT assessment and summing up.

MAKING THE TREATMENT MODEL EXPLICIT

Finally, the therapist should provide the patient with some idea of what will be offered, including the fact that treatment will be time limited. Depending upon the information gathered at the interview and on the clinical picture of the larynx, the therapist will decide whether to focus treatment towards direct voice therapy or through cognitive behaviour therapy. Frequently there will be an element of both, or the therapist will begin by directing treatment through voice therapy. This often makes a lot of sense because several of the techniques used in voice therapy are employed by the therapist using cognitive behavioural therapy. Such techniques would include body awareness, an appreciation of tension sites, particularly tension in the vocal tract, and relaxation and centred breathing. The extent of the explanation of cognitive behaviour therapy at this stage is likely to be determined by the priority that the therapist plans to give this in treatment. It may be that it will not be the dominant focus of therapy initially. Whenever the time is appropriate to explain the use of cognitive behaviour therapy this can also be quite explicit. Many cognitive behaviour therapists will give the patient a brief summary of the treatment model and the implications for their treatment. Since, in the majority of cases of psychogenic voice disorder, there will be stressful interpersonal relationships, the therapist will probably emphasise the role of autonomic arousal in situations of conflict, will mention the value of using anxiety reduction techniques and of training in assertiveness or the expression of views and will then move on to describing the value of collecting current data and how this can be done by keeping a daily record of such things as stressful events, thoughts, emotions, behavioural reactions and voice quality. It may also be necessary to explain the relevance of events in our past and how they have shaped reactions to situations today, and then to explain that the techniques we have just described will be used to change habitual responses. In presenting this information the therapist also conveys something of the collaborative nature of treatment.

A SUMMARY OF HOW TO CONCLUDE THE INTERVIEW

- Offer the patient the opportunity to add anything important. Invite questions.
- Acknowledge when the interview has been emotionally demanding. Thank the patient for their participation.
- Provide the patient with a psychological or cognitive behavioural explanation for their symptoms.
- Reflect and provide a tentative hypothesis. Explain voice production and vocal strain. Summarise and select important causal factors. Offer a tentative interpretation connecting the laryngeal muscle tension and functioning of the vocal folds with the psychological causal features. This will help the patient to understand their experiences and in so doing reassure the patient of their mental health.
- Make the treatment model explicit; this is likely to combine attention to the function of the voice and to the psychological features. Highlight the problem-solution focus and the role of client collaboration and self-help.
- Outline a time-limited treatment contract.

WORKING WITHIN A FRAMEWORK OF CLINICAL SUPERVISION

The position we are taking is that speech and language therapists may adopt a CBT approach both within their assessment and subsequent therapy and that this will enhance the quality and effectiveness of the intervention. The therapist's bias towards symptomatic therapy or CBT will be governed by the patient's individual needs and

Table 4.4: Standard voice case history form with psychosocial 'screening' prompts

Name: d.o.b.:   age:

Address:

Phone:

Occupation:

Referred by: date:

Next ENT appointment:

Date of Assessment:

Patient Information

Onset and History of Voice Problem

Any previous voice problem/voice therapy

Description of present problem

Sensations in vocal tract

Reaction to dysphonia. (*'How do you feel about your voice problem? Has it stopped you doing anything?'*)

Variation of the problem

Consistency

Better situations

Worse Situations

Description of vocal use

Work, hobbies, sport, leisure time

('Do you have much time for yourself and do you use this time? What sort of relaxation do you do? Do you sing? Would you say you relax well or do you find you never sit down?')

Related Medical History

Previous illnesses/surgery

Drug or hormone therapy

Present health

URT [asthma, bronchitis, allergies, etc.]

Smoking/drinking

('How do you feel in general?' 'How are your energy levels?')

Associated Factors
Sleep pattern *('Has this changed recently?' 'What things keep you awake at night?')*

Appetite/weight

Headache/migraine

Breathlessness *('What might bring this on?' 'Can you think of a specific time when this has happened?')*

Panic attacks *'What was going on in your life the last time this happened?'*

('Do you think you are a worrier?')

Observations of Patient

Tension sites [reported and observed]

Face

Jaw

Neck/Shoulder

General Body

Posture and examination of laryngeal musculature

Perceptual Voice Assessment

Objective Voice Measures

Personal History

Family Tree:

Married ..... Co-habiting..... Single ..... Separated ..... Divorced ..... Widowed ..... *('Who is at home with you?' 'Do you have children?' 'Who is the main bread winner?' 'Are you/ your partner in stable employment?')*

Children – at home/away *('Who is the main carer?')*
Family relationships: *('Are there others that you care for?')*
('How would you describe your relationships with your immediate family?')

Significant Life Events

[Bereavements, losses, moves, changes in relationship, changes at work, etc.]
('Have there been any significant changes in your life over the past couple of years or so? For instance, have you had any bereavements or have you had any changes in your job or at home?')

Events Immediately Preceding the Dysphonia

('Can you think back to when your voice trouble started. Was there anything going on at that time that might have upset you?')

Relationship Conflicts/Expressing Views

('Is there anyone at home or at work whom you have been having problems with, such as your partner, children, someone in the family or your boss or colleagues?' 'Have you had trouble expressing your feelings to these people?' 'How good are you at telling people what you want or how you feel?' 'How would your family describe you?')

Balancing Responsibilities and Commitments

('Whom would you turn to for your support?' 'How good are you at asking for support?' 'Do you take time for yourself?')

Health and Finances

('Have you been concerned about your health or the health of your family, or about your career or your finances?')

Patient's View of Voice Problem

('Have you any idea about what might be causing the voice problem?')

Clinical Impressions

Diagnosis or Formulation and Action Plan

Further examples of psychosocial prompts can be found in the text of Chapter 4.

their readiness to explore the emotions behind their voice. Combining symptomatic voice therapy and CBT is explored further in the following chapter. At all times we do advocate that the speech and language therapist works within a framework of supervision supported by a clinical psychologist skilled in CBT or a specialist practitioner in CBT. There may indeed be instances when the speech and language therapist recognises, from the complexities of the case, the need to refer the patient on for management by the clinical psychologist, rather than to work with supervision.

SUMMARY

- A voice case history is incomplete if it does not include sufficient assessment of psychosocial health. We advocate that some psychosocial screening should be incorporated into all voice assessments whilst full psychosocial assessment is reserved for a minority of patients. Guidance is given to help the SLT determine when a screening or full psychosocial assessment is indicated (pp. 59–61).
- Understanding the common aetiological features of PVD helps the SLT to focus case history taking. These common aetiological features are described and their implications for a more complete psychosocial assessment of the patient are summarised.
- When conducting a psychosocial interview cognitive behaviour counselling skills are recommended. These were previously explored in Chapter 3 and are reviewed briefly in this chapter for the SLT (pp. 69–70). Although many of these skills will be familiar to the experienced SLT working with voice disorders, they

can be acquired or extended through postgraduate training and through working within a framework of clinical supervision with a clinical psychologist.
- A framework is provided that allows for psychosocial history taking within a voice case history. The standard voice case history is extended to either include psychosocial screening questions or extended for a comprehensive psychosocial assessment. There is discussion and example of the areas that a SLT might include in a psychosocial assessment.
- The chapter offers a standard voice case history proforma that includes psychosocial screening prompts.

5 Symptomatic Voice Therapy Approaches

Voice therapy techniques are essential to the successful management of psychogenic voice disorders, whether the patient presents with aphonia or dysphonia. In only a few cases will the therapist find the patient resistant to such interventions although, such resistance in itself can contribute information to the diagnosis. In Chapter 1 we presented our classification system for both psychogenic dysphonia and aphonia and discussed those patients most likely to respond well to a combined approach of symptomatic voice therapy and CBT, namely the Type 2 (cognitive behavioural) patient group. Andersson and Schalen 1998, note that cognitive behavioural therapy, as a treatment in isolation for psychogenic voice disorder, is usually unsatisfactory but when combined with voice exercises is effective in the majority of cases. We would certainly say that this is the case for the Type 2 (cognitive behavioural) patient group. Type 3 (psychogenic-habituated) patients, where the precipitating stressors or conflicts are diminished or resolved, are also likely to do well using symptomatic voice therapy and are likely to require little in the way of psychological therapy. Cognitive behaviour therapy for these patients is likely to take a preventative stance, acknowledging that although precipitating factors may have resolved, predisposing factors such as the patients' schema and coping strategies may make them vulnerable to recurrence. In contrast, the Type 1 (classical hysterical) patient, who is most likely to be resistant to the interventions of the SLT using symptomatic voice therapy with or without a combination of CBT, will require referral on to a psychologist or psychiatrist. Table 5.1 outlines the typical management approach that we would recommend for Types 1–3 and Chapter 6 expands on this.

In Chapter 4 we discussed the importance of a detailed ENT examination before commencing therapeutic input. We reiterate here the need for the therapist to refer back to ENT any patient for whom the voice presentation/history and ENT diagnosis do not concur.

For reasons we will explain, the initial approach taken by the therapist will depend largely on whether the patient presents with aphonia or dysphonia, rather than the classification of their psychogenic disorder. We would argue, along with others that the dysphonic patient, rather than the aphonic, can present the greater challenge, because of the need to modify the vocal gesture rather than simply effect a dramatic return of voice. (Boone & McFarlane 2000; Mathieson 2001.) However, the voice therapist who is already experienced in treating muscle misuse dysphonia will find many techniques equally appropriate for the psychogenic dysphonic. We will outline our approach for both aphonics and dysphonics separately.

Table 5.1: Recommended treatment approaches for psychogenic dysphonia/aphonia
$\sqrt{}$ = recommended

Category of Psychogenic Dysphonia/Aphonia	Voice Therapy	CBT	Psychiatry
Type 1 (classical hysterical)	$\sqrt{}$ Diagnostic only	x	$\sqrt{}$
Type 2 (cognitive-behavioural)	$\sqrt{}$	$\sqrt{}$	x
Type 3 (psychogenic-habituated)	$\sqrt{}$	$\sqrt{}$ Preventing recurrance	x

MANAGING THE APHONIC PATIENT

PREPARATION FOR RESTORING THE VOICE

Restoration of the voice should be the primary goal for the therapist's first session with an *aphonic* patient. There are a number of reasons why this approach is recommended. First, the majority of patients' voices will be easily restored with this approach (Baker 1998; Boone & McFarlane 2000; Mathieson 2001) as their psychological profile will be that of the Type 2 or 3. A quick resolution of the voice eliminates the frustration and handicap associated with voice loss, and precipitating and perpetuating psychological factors can then be more readily explored. Second, the longer the patient uses the faulty voice set, the more habitualised the patterns become and the harder it will be to effect return of voice using voice therapy techniques (Tucker 1987; Mathieson 2001). Third, the patient who identifies early on that the voice problem may be due to conflicts and stress may be less receptive to guided symptom removal. Such patients may become more aware of the therapeutic process and thus more guarded in how they participate in symptomatic techniques, potentially reducing their ability to benefit. Finally, an aphonic patient's response to symptomatic voice therapy forms part of the diagnostic process and in itself helps guide the clinician to distinguish between the patient with a Type 1 *vs* a Type 2 or 3 disorder. The Type 1 patient will typically *resist* the therapist's attempts to restore voice and/or demonstrate an inappropriate response to the restoration of voice, e.g. passivity or denial, possibly leaving the therapist feeling dissatisfied or frustrated or even murderous!

Voice restoration should be anticipated in the majority of cases and wherever possible the patients should leave the clinic after the initial session with voice, or with the belief that they are now capable of normal communication. The therapist would be wise to schedule a minimum of an hour long initial appointment to ensure there is adequate time to develop the voice adequately.

The therapist needs to adopt an authoritative, clear and confident approach when introducing the patient to symptomatic voice therapy approaches. We would go as far as to suggest that the success of treatment rests as much with the patient's faith in the clinician's ability to 'cure' as in the selection of treatment techniques themselves. As early as 1969, this style of delivery was fittingly described by Brodnitz as 'an air of unhurried persuasiveness'. Aronson (1990a, p. 323) refers to the 'clinician's finesse' and the therapist may indeed feel that he/she is employing great mental and physical energy throughout such a session. Employing such a style does not obviate the need to remain sensitive to the patient's verbal and non-verbal cues, and we will describe later occasions when the need for a gentler approach becomes evident.

It is important to establish expectations from the start, i.e. that the therapist believes the prognosis to be very good and that with full attention from the patient the problem will resolve. The therapist needs to have a number of treatment techniques up his/her sleeve and to move calmly, yet swiftly from one to another until the most positive vocalisation is heard. Although an initial session with an aphonic usually instills a degree of anxious expectation in the therapist, it is important not to convey anxiety or to allow the patient to feel failure if voice is not facilitated immediately. It is possible to prepare the patient for this approach with very simple explanation, e.g. '*I am going to take you through some simple exercises to explore your problem further. When we have tried these I can explain to you what I think will help and why. You may find some of these exercises easier than others.*'

It is interesting to the authors that Type 2 patients respond so positively to a symptomatic voice therapy approach in the early stages of treatment, when assessment of these patients so clearly demonstrates that they are suppressing emotional conflicts and experiencing associated anxiety. At the same time and as we have outlined above, we believe firmly that the style in which the therapist conducts that very first session can be a key to successfully guiding the patient towards voice restoration. We have speculated that this authoritative style of delivery is itself offering the Type 2 patients a position of safety and control that enables them to lower their defenses and literally 'speak out' and voice.

VOICE THERAPY TREATMENT TECHNIQUES

FACILITATIVE PHONATORY METHODS

Those symptomatic voice therapy techniques most frequently used by the authors are summarised in Table 5.2. Voice is most easily initiated using vegetative phonatory behaviours. Behaviours such as throat clearing, laughing, grunting on a shoulder shrug, coughing and inspiratory voicing elicit vocal fold adduction as part of the vegetative, or more primitive functions of the larynx and as such are removed from the communicative functions of the voice. As techniques, they provide a window into first, demonstrating to the patient that the larynx is capable of generating normal sound and second, providing the first step from which to develop voice. We have found that in some cases a more active routine of body movements and strenuous exercise, e.g. stretching, reaching, arm swings and jumping combined with vegetative voicing, aids the release of breath and voice. In these instances the therapist needs to guide the patient through a range of body movements encouraging the patient to copy his/her movements and voice. The therapist needs to provide confident and dramatic modelling with movements and vocalisations that will be bigger

Table 5.2: Voice therapy treatment techniques for the aphonic patient

Facilitative phonatory techniques	Cough/throat clear
	Laughing
	Expiratory 'hmm'
	Gargling
	Shoulder shrugging
	Inspiratory voicing
	Lip and tongue trills
	Vocal fry/creaky voice
	Exhalation with manual vibration of lower rib cage and diaphragmatic region
	Body movement with vocalisation
Sound extension techniques	Glottal onsets with exaggerated intonation e.g. 'óh òh'
	Vowel shaping
	Fricative sound prolongation
	Chanting
Relaxation methods	Laryngeal manipulation/ manual relaxation
	Relaxation with imagery
	Systematic relaxation techniques
Additional techniques	Masking – Lombard effect.
	Biofeedback
Therapist skills	Authoritative, confident style
	Generous encouragement
	Quick successive treatment steps
	Physiological explanations early on in treatment
	Sensitivity and responsiveness to the patient's verbal and non-verbal cues.

and louder than the patients to allow them to feel comfortable. Although this approach may at first seem most suited to children we have found it to be successful with a range of ages.

Direct manipulation of the laryngeal mechanism (Lieberman in Harris et al. 1998) can be effective in releasing tense postures and thus freeing up the voice, e.g. releasing the tight, high larynx or closed cricothyroid visor. Such hands-on techniques may also be useful before eliciting voice. Manipulation with simultaneous explanation by the SLT serves to highlight the role that muscle tension plays in maintaining the aphonia and psychologically gives the patient permission to let go as well as allowing the patient time to develop trust in the therapist.

The therapist is advised not to draw attention to the patient's initial voice attempts, as this may well inhibit the release of the voice. It is better to work steadily through a range of techniques allowing the voice to develop without showing surprise or excitement over its return but instead an implicit acceptance.

MASKING

The authors recommend that the therapist perform vocal tasks simultaneously and at a louder volume than the patient. The use of auditory masking to produce a reflexive vocal response was introduced in 1911 by Lombard and is known as the Lombard effect. By masking the patient's own attempts, their auditory feedback is diminished. This serves both to block the habitualised feedback mechanisms and to reduce the patient's self-consciousness and thus his/her chances of regression. The therapist can gradually remove his/her vocal masking as the patient moves into a new vocal set. Boone (1977) advocates using headphones with a masking noise while the patient reads aloud, to reflexively establish voicing. Baker (1998) describes using a keyboard and singing loudly with a patient to reduce auditory feedback at this critical stage in treatment (p. 534).

Once a normal vocal sound is produced and heard by the patient, they can be encouraged to sustain that note on vowels of differing height and then into chanted phrases, etc. The therapist may need to be firm and directive at this stage to prevent the patient opting out and reverting back to an aphonic phonatory pattern, e.g.'*No. Use your strong voice now.*' Sometimes this may mean prolonging the appointment by 10–15 minutes to ensure the voice is established and that it can be used in speaking, loud voicing and even singing. The patient's voice may not sound or feel entirely normal and the therapist should reinforce that it will settle over the coming days as the muscles readjust.

SOUND EXTENSION TECHNIQUES AND DEVELOPMENT OF THE VOICE

The therapist should develop the voice quickly through a series of sound extension tasks and into conversation within this initial session. The patient should be encouraged to converse not only with the therapist but where possible with relatives, clinic staff, etc., before they leave, as this can rapidly instill confidence. This behavioural bridging to people or situations outside of the clinic room is important so that the patient's self-construct is that of a normal speaker and not a voiceless person. The therapist may direct the patient to phone home from the clinic, using the new voice or speak to clinic staff.

Some therapists may choose to take a more nurturing route to generalisation, identifying with the patient safe communication partners with whom to use the new voice initially, gradually increasing the exposure to less safe situations. In the majority of cases where voice is restored in the initial session, it will be important to arrange for a follow-up session, ideally within a one to two week time frame. This second session allows the therapist both to support the patient's maintenance of voicing and to develop the assessment of precipitating and maintaining psychological factors. Once completed the therapist will have a clearer idea as to the need to incorporate psychological methods into the treatment programme, and to discover whether they have the requisite skills to work through these with the patient. In the case of a Type 3 patient, where the initial stressors have resolved, this assessment may be quite brief, but some reflection with this patient as to the causes of the aphonia may offer insight and closure to the initial episode.

Lydia's case provides an example of a Type 3 (psychogenic-habituated) aphonic patient with a quick recovery of voice achieved through the use of symptomatic voice therapy techniques. Although there was clearly a traumatic event and associated emotional conflict associated with the onset of the voice difficulty, some six months previously, psychological screening suggested there were no unresolved issues for the patient. However, psychosocial questioning around the 3 Ps did raise the patient's own awareness of her tendency to worry and thus heightened her receptiveness to relaxation techniques as a mechanism for dealing with symptoms of stress.

For the full case history see Chapter 10, pp. 200–2.

USING BIOFEEDBACK

In some cases, the patient may not achieve full restoration of voice in the initial session, although glimpses of the normal/near normal voice will have been heard. It is vital that these voicing episodes be identified and reinforced and here, biofeedback methods may be of value. The patient who lacks body awareness or has become detached from his/her laryngeal mechanism may be assisted by feeling the phonatory vibrations with their hand at the level of the thyroid cartilage or by seeing the vibrations using instrumentation such as the electrolaryngograph. Audio feedback may provide encouragement for some patients but very soon, as with all voice therapy, patients should be encouraged to report on their own sensations of voicing. The SLT can then adjust the vocal pattern according to what they observe and hear.

POSITIVE REINFORCEMENT AND SUGGESTION

The patient who achieves only some voice in the first session should be reassured that normal voice 'will return', with the therapist making the suggestion that this may happen that same evening or across the week. '*Your voice will return but the muscles that have become tensed and tight need a little time. I would expect you to hear (more) voice later today or tomorrow.*' This positive and confident approach is crucial to achieving eventual success. The patient may be asked to call at an agreed time to report on return of voice after practising a few simple exercises. A follow-up appointment or successive appointments should be scheduled to follow on as soon as possible, ideally within a week. In such cases where return of voice is gradual, it may be very appropriate to combine symptomatic voice therapy with psychological assessment and management as outlined in previous chapters.

A SLOWER APPROACH

The traditional approach to managing the aphonic patient, i.e. that of facilitating a return of voice in the first session, may for a minority of patients be too rapid a therapeutic process and one which then makes it difficult to follow through a psychological approach, despite there being clear psychological signs at interview. The therapist will need to be sensitive to the patient's verbal and non-verbal responses during the first session and be flexible if necessary to how far he/she leads the patient to achieving early restoration of voice. It is important to take pauses during explanations and between tasks, giving time for the therapist to judge the patient's responses to episodes of voicing. Patients who are not psychologically ready to speak out may plateau quite quickly in a session having achieved moments of normal or near normal voice. This does not in itself suggest they are a Type 1 patient as they do not display other distinguishing features such as *la belle indifference* (see p. 8). Such patients may indeed fit the profile of a Type 2 psychogenic disorder and be motivated for voice therapy and frustrated with their voice loss. These patients simply require a more non-pressured and supportive approach incorporating a more considered psychological approach alongside voice therapy techniques. This may be the case with some children and adolescents. With all patients it is essential to be sensitive to the emotional origins of the voice loss as well as to the emotional challenge of its return. In facilitating the return of voice the therapist must avoid exposing the patient's vulnerability.

Anne is an aphonic young woman who achieved a rapid return of voice through symptomatic therapy, but where it was difficult to follow through a psychological approach, despite a very obvious need. Initial presentation would suggest the profile of a Type 2 psychogenic voice disorder although full psychosocial assessment was not completed. The patient's affect and family dynamics in the initial session all left the clinician highly suspicious that the patient was being emotionally abused. A rapid return of voice or 'cure', seemingly left the patient with no overt reason to return for further sessions.

For the full case history see Chapter 10, pp. 189–91.

Finally we must consider the patient who does not respond positively to symptomatic therapy techniques within the first few sessions and who fits our category of Type 1 patients. These patients will exhibit other tell-tale signs such as the detachment as previously described in Chapter 1. The SLT should refer these patients to psychiatry for further assessment, confirmation of the diagnosis and therapeutic input if appropriate. The process of referral on to psychiatry can be challenging, but the authors believe that it is important for the therapist to be overt about the fact that he/she believes the problem to originate from psychological processes and that these are beyond the skill-base of a SLT to manage. The case study of Diana in Chapter 10, p. 175–8 illustrates this process of Type 1 closure more explicitly. Although the psychiatrist may also be able to offer little that can facilitate improvement in this patient group, it is important to have the diagnosis confirmed and to have excluded other formulations (see Chapter 9 for further discussion).

James is a Type 2 (cognitive behavioural) aphonic teenager. His case identifies a complex psychosocial history with significant emotional factors.

The patient was treated successfully primarily using symptomatic voice therapy. Detailed psychological assessment enabled the therapist to empathise effectively and to identify the value of including support and ego-boosting within the management programme.

For the full case history see Chapter 10, pp. 185–9.

There are other factors which may indicate the likelihood of a poor outcome with symptomatic speech therapy with/without psychological input. These are outlined in Table 5.3.

The voice therapy techniques we have described for the aphonic patient are not exhaustive and the clinician may identify additional techniques used with other patient groups that are of benefit. To some extent the therapist can capitalise on his/her own creativity and personal style.

Treating an aphonic patient is both challenging and rewarding for the speech and language therapist. There are few other such dramatic sessions for both therapist and patient and the therapist should be prepared for a variety of responses to the return of voice. Many patients feel overwhelmed and may be tearful or unable to verbally express their feelings immediately. They must be given time to recognise their emotions and to express their feelings. Some patients fear that others may perceive their rapid recovery as an indication of their malingering and need support in explaining their recovery to family and friends. As we have shown, the return of voice may mark only the start of the therapeutic process and the relationship developed between

Table 5.3: Negative prognostic factors in treatment of psychogenic aphonia/dysphonia

- Detachment towards/lack of distress at dysphonic/aphonic symptoms (*la belle indifference*)
- Dysphonia/aphonia of long duration
- Persistent symptoms with no periods of normal/near normal voice
- Experience of previous unsuccessful treatment programmes
- Resistance to idea of influencing psychological factors
- Primary *and* secondary gains identified from the history
- No confidence in therapist's ability to restore voice
- No reassured that concomitant symptoms e.g. globus, cough, are not due to medical problem
- Poor motivation to participate in treatment
- Signs of psychiatric disorder (see Chapter 9)

Adapted from Morrison and Rammage 1993

therapist and patient in the initial session is paramount to the overall effectiveness of the healing process.

MANAGING THE DYSPHONIC PATIENT

PREPARATION FOR RESTORING THE VOICE

The larger number of patients with a psychogenic voice disorder will present with *dysphonia* rather than *aphonia*. We would advocate the need for a more gradual approach to voice restoration for the dysphonic patient than the aphonic described previously. In the case of the dysphonic we recommend that voice therapy techniques are best introduced once the interviewing process is completed. Except for a small number of Type 1 patients, dysphonic patients with a psychogenic disorder, tend to fit the Type 2 and Type 3 categories. As we discussed in Chapter 1, their vocal profile may be very diverse. Forced and strained voices, ventricular band voicing, falsetto, breathy voice, etc. may all have an underlying psychogenic cause, and mucosal changes to the larynx as a result of utilising a tense phonatory pattern may also occur. It is thus impossible to diagnose the psychogenic dysphonic from perceptual or laryngeal examination alone. It will only be through a diagnostic interview that incorporates a comprehensive psychosocial case history and voice assessment, such as that described in Chapter 4, that an adequate working hypothesis can be formulated.

In Chapter 4, we outlined the areas to consider within the psychosocial case history and discussed the importance of adopting a flexible approach to the interviewing process. Although the aim should be to complete the psychological screening questions as early on as possible, not all patients will feel able to disclose personal information at this stage and it may be that issues of an emotional nature emerge gradually. Some patients will disclose everything straight away, with little effort on the part of the therapist, and others not until symptomatic therapy has been commenced. In the latter case, the therapist will need to negotiate with the patient the need to briefly step back from symptomatic work until the significance of the personal information is ascertained.

Once the degree of psychological influence is established and the type of psychogenic dysphonia clarified, the clinician will wish to negotiate or review the type of treatment package to be provided. The patient needs to understand the degree to which symptomatic voice therapy alone can resolve their problems. Type 1 patients are unlikely to benefit from voice therapy approaches and should be referred to psychiatry as early on as possible, although the full profile of the Type 1 may only become totally clear after some voice therapy techniques are trialed. In the case of the Type 3 dysphonic patient, where precipitating and perpetuating psychological factors are largely resolved, it will be most appropriate to work using those vocal function techniques used with other hyperfunctional patients and a good resolution of symptoms should be anticipated. Some of these techniques are outlined later on in this chapter. As the Type 3 group of patients achieve resolution of their vocal symptoms, it may become appropriate to incorporate a few simple cognitive behavioural techniques into the management programme, e.g. systematic relaxation, in order to minimise the likelihood of recurrence in the future.

In contrast to the Type 3 group, we would suggest that long-term resolution in the case of Type 2 patients is most likely where they select a package of treatment that combines symptomatic voice therapy and a CBT approach. It is the role of the therapist to supply the options for the type of treatment approach, i.e. symptomatic therapy alone with a chance of recurrence or symptomatic therapy and CBT with a greater chance of long-term resolution; this assumption is supported by the work of Butcher et al. 1987 and Andersson and Schalen 1998. It should be the patient who elects which route to take once informed of these options and anticipated outcomes. Butcher and Cavalli (1998) outline a typical case in which the patient, Fran, achieved *control* of her dysphonia and laryngeal symptoms following five voice therapy sessions. However, it was felt that long-term *resolution* would be more likely if she could be helped to develop strategies for managing her considerable burden of responsibility and over-commitment and to resolve her conflict over speaking out in significant emotional relationships. Following 16 sessions of psychological treatment, a cognitive behavioural therapy approach enabled her to develop assertiveness skills, control symptoms of anxiety and reduce her burden of responsibility. She felt empowered to take control of her own life stressors and concluded therapy at a point where she had been able to test out her own ability to control her symptoms.

Fran had attended the voice clinic with a thick health record, which detailed a number of assessments by other health care specialities. Tests for respiratory and cardiac symptoms had all resulted in a clean bill of health. On reflection it is clear that her symptoms of palpitations and difficulty breathing were related to high levels of anxiety. Her dysphonia was a conversion of suppressed anxiety, which was identified early on in speech and language therapy sessions. Fran was offered two different therapy contracts: the first to offer symptom relief in the form of traditional voice therapy, and the second to offer longer term resolution of her dysphonia and associated symptoms. This is frequently a successful way to present the therapy contract.

The patient's ability to make an informed choice of management programme will be facilitated by a clear explanation of the problem. The SLT must offer a succinct and comprehensive explanation for the patient's symptoms before engaging them in exercises that improve the vocal gesture and develop voice production. This stage in management is discussed in more detail in Chapter 4. We would agree with others (Baker 1998; Boone & McFarlane 2000; Mathieson 2001) that a physiological explanation based around what the patient is doing, i.e. '*Your vocal muscles are tense and are thus preventing the vocal folds from coming together*', rather than a psychological one, is important until the SLT is confident to have classified the patient's psychological profile. Typically however, Type 2 patients will volunteer a number of stressors early on in the process and it is possible to offer this group of patients a combined physiological-psychological explanation of the impact of the life events and stressors on the voice, although always still attributing blame to the muscles and not the person. For example, '*You have told me about a number of things that make me think that you have had quite a bit of stress to deal with recently. We know that stress can make the muscles in our body tighten up and sometimes they find it difficult to relax again if the stress continues for a while or is quite significant. Our throat muscles are particularly vulnerable to stress and when they tighten it can alter the way our voice sounds. I am wondering whether this could be the explanation for your voice difficulty. What do you feel about this?'* Baker (1998), in her presentation of two complex cases of psychogenic aphonia, highlights the importance of framing the explanation for recovery in terms that lower the patient's defenses and allow them to relax sufficiently to explore a psychological explanation for their problem. She outlines the importance of determination, adaptability and creative cunning on the part of the therapist.

There will be a few Type 2 cases where the patient will not be ready to accept a psychological approach and the therapist will need to be flexible in using voice-focused sessions as a way to establish the trusting relationship required for the patient to gain acceptance. Such acceptance may also come as these patients reach a plateau in vocal function. When agreeing the format of the treatment package the patient should feel that they can review their decision at any time.

Sue presents the case of a Type 2 dysphonic woman and demonstrates the importance of the psychological interview in helping the patient have a full insight of the psychological conflicts underpinning the dysphonia, thereby facilitating both a return to normal voice and a decision to work through the underlying conflicts in her separation from her husband.

For the full case history see Chapter 10, pp. 191–4.

VOICE THERAPY TREATMENT TECHNIQUES

The primary aim of this part of the treatment package will be to 'free the voice'. As with many patients there will be a stage, early on in the treatment programme, where it may be difficult to predict the particular vocal technique(s) or method which will be most effective in achieving a free voice. The concepts of probe testing (Koschkee & Rammage 1997) and diagnostic therapy, are useful here. The SLT may wish to move quite rapidly between a series of tasks/behaviours before identifying the most appropriate. If they are not careful the patient may feel confused and lose confidence in the clinician's ability for voice restoration. At the outset therefore, and in the same way as with the aphonic patient, it is important to explain to the patient that he/she will be led through a series of tasks that will allow the therapist and patient to learn more about the patient's voice. The therapist will need to reassure the patient that by the end of the session the techniques for help will be clarified.

The following techniques are in no way exhaustive but have been considered by the authors to be most helpful in freeing the voice of the psychogenic dysphonic. The reader is referred to key texts elsewhere for detailed descriptions of appropriate methods and techniques.

RELAXATION

It will frequently be appropriate to incorporate relaxation techniques into the voice therapy programme of the psychogenic dysphonic as well as the aphonic. The value of relaxation as part of a CBT approach is discussed in Chapter 3. For the patient experiencing dysphonia associated with high stress levels and raised muscle tension, relaxation techniques may serve two purposes. The first objective is to establish a kinaesthetic model of relaxed musculature, which acts as a baseline from which the patient can monitor excessive tension (Mathieson 2001). In this way, the patient learns to use relaxation techniques to release body tensions and begin to free the breath and the voice. Second, if used at the start of a session, relaxation strategies may establish a state of readiness and responsiveness from which the patient can best learn. It should be noted that the choice of technique is very important and some patients may feel very guarded and exposed if asked to close their eyes and lie in a supine position. The clinician must therefore be skilled in a number of different techniques.

SLTs trained in hypnosis may also find this a useful adjunct to therapy. In the authors' experience, hypnosis can be used in a treatment plan to help facilitate a return of voice through deep relaxation, reducing inhibition and resistance and providing a strong suggestion of normal voice and ego-strengthening. It is not the authors' approach to use hypnosis as a therapy in itself but to use it selectively when a resolution is slow and provided that the patient is willing or has indeed requested hypnosis.

FACILITATING TECHNIQUES

Techniques such as the yawn-sigh (Boone 1977) and Froeshel's chewing methods (1948) aim to establish a vocal gesture from which the patient can experience free voice. The yawn-sigh technique elicits pharyngeal widening and a lowered larynx thus extending the vocal tract length and facilitating vocal resonance for the patient with a tight, high laryngeal posture (Boone & McFarlane 1993). Others, such as Linklater (1976) and Shewell (2000), outline a more complete approach to freeing the voice that incorporates work both on the body and the breath. Manual techniques for reducing tension of the laryngeal mechanism (Lieberman in Harris et al. 1998) may also benefit, by reducing discomfort and freeing the voice in a similar way to the approach described for the aphonic patient.

SPEECH-BREATHING AND VOCAL FUNCTION EXERCISES

Breathing techniques and vocal function exercises aimed at initiating a smooth vocal onset, reducing articulatory tension and deconstricting the laryngeal and supraglottic gesture are described in detail by other authors (Morrison & Rammage 1993; Yanagisawa et al. 1996; Andersson & Schalen 1998; Harris et al. 1998; Boone &

McFarlane 2000; Mathieson 2001; Thyme-Frokjaer & Frokjaer-Jensen 2001) and will not be outlined here although they may well be incorporated into the treatment plan of the dysphonic patient where the vocal gesture restored early on in treatment is not totally free due to habitualised patterns.

BIOFEEDBACK

As with the aphonic patient, some dysphonics will benefit from visualising their voice production, e.g. with the use of acoustic signals provided from instrumentation such as electrolaryngography (Fourcin 1986). In Chapter 4 we discussed the potential for using laryngoscopic feedback to aid patients understanding their problem at a diagnostic level. Nasendoscopy (examination of the larynx through a flexible endoscope while the patient is awake) is increasingly being used by therapists as an adjunct to therapy and may have a valuable role in helping the patient achieve the target vocal gestures (Rattenbury et al. 2004). As with all patients, the therapist should be selective as to which psychogenic patient may be a suitable candidate for this approach, remembering that this area may be particularly sensitive for some. However, results can be quite rapid and allow the therapist to move quickly on to sound extension work once the patient has a kinaesthetic model for the free voice.

COMBINING VOICE THERAPY AND CBT

Speech and language therapists may be cautious about combining CBT approaches with symptomatic voice therapy with the arguments that it extends the length of the patient's treatment and/or that they are not skilled to do so. With regard to the first point, we would argue that a combined psychological and symptomatic treatment approach is in the long-term most cost-effective and time-efficient for many patients with psychogenic voice disorder. White, Deary and Wilson (1997) support this viewpoint, noting that although the initial response of psychogenic dysphonia patients to voice therapy is good, a small number fail to respond to treatment and there is a high relapse rate in those who initially respond well. The authors have shown that CBT approaches can facilitate vocal improvement in 50% of psychogenic voice disordered patients found previously not to respond to intensive symptomatic voice therapy combined with client-centred counselling approaches (Butcher et al. 1987). In a recent randomised control pilot study, CBT-enhanced voice therapy provided by a speech and language therapist was shown to improve outcomes for dysphonic patients when compared to patients having voice therapy alone (Daniilidou 2006).

Unlike traditional psychotherapies, CBT offers a time-limited approach usually between eight and 20 sessions. It is usual to offer an initial treatment contract of six to eight sessions and to review progress at the end of this intense time period of approximately two months. The time between later sessions is usually extended to allow patients to develop confidence in their ability to take control of their own symptoms and to function independently from the therapist's support. This approach will be familiar to most speech and language therapists and sits well in the modern times of treatment contracts and packages of care.

The number of sessions required will of course depend on the complexity of the specific case. We have found that the majority of patients with a psychogenic disorder require 3–16 sessions. A prospective and longitudinal study of 30 dysphonic patients by Andersson and Schalen (1998) found that 63% of patients received a maximum of five therapy sessions, lasting between 45 and 60 minutes and a further 20% received more than ten sessions. Their approach combined voice therapy and cognitive behavioural techniques. Follow-up between one and eight years later suggested 88% of patients had maintained progress. These results compare favourably with timescales reported elsewhere for different patient groups. Lockhart, Paton and Pearson (1997) calculated treatment timescales for different patient categories in a cross-centre study. The average number of sessions used to treat patients with vocal strain and oedema was eight sessions and nodules and ventricular overreaction required an average of seven sessions, although all categories showed considerable variation with ranges between two and 16 sessions. These authors had a separate group of patients they classified as psychogenic, for which no timescales were reported due to the diversity of the group. Some patients will require longer treatment contracts. Baker (1998), who is a highly-skilled SLT with additional family therapy training, describes a complex case of a Type 1 conversion, requiring 24 sessions of advanced psychological support combined with voice therapy and demonstrates that, without this level of input, resolution was unsuccessful. The total treatment package for Fran, outlined on p. 98, comprised 21 sessions (Butcher & Cavalli 1998) and combined the skills of the clinical psychologist and a speech and language therapist.

In answering concerns from the therapist about requisite skills we take the stance that speech and language therapists are well-placed to acquire skills in CBT and that this can be done through postgraduate training and/or co-working and clinical supervision with a clinical therapist. It is in line with mental health work that professionals such as SLTs should be trained and empowered to have these extended skills to support a wider population and, in order to provide the best resolution for PVD, we would argue this is essential.

CONCLUDING THE THERAPY CONTRACT

Knowing that treatment is time-limited can increase patient motivation and this, as well as gradually extending the time between later sessions, can be a factor that reduces patient dependence. Patients should be reminded how many sessions remain and allowed to explore their feelings about concluding treatment. They should be offered opportunities to rehearse their new skills, thus building confidence in their independent self-help.

The majority of patients will conclude treatment having resolved their dysphonia and having gained sufficient skills and insight to independently manage future challenging life experiences. Some may experience one or more episodes of dysphonia for which they require additional support. Usually no more than one or two sessions is sufficient to review the situation and revisit helpful strategies. For this reason the client should be informed that another assessment and treatment contract can be arranged if a crisis occurs at any time in the future.

As with any other type of treatment, there will be patients for whom a combined CBT-SLT approach is not suited. The reasons for this are varied (Butcher et al. 1987). Some patients, despite support, find the requirement for self-help too challenging. As with a traditional voice therapy approach, the patient must be motivated to fully participate in treatment sessions and also to follow a programme of exercises and tasks at home. Many patients already experience very complicated lives and support is required to enable them to see the benefits of taking on another challenge, namely that of attending appointments and home rehearsal. Some patients may decide that it is not the right time to embark on treatment. Providing this decision is informed and communicated to all relevant professionals involved in the patient's care, future appropriate management of the patient's dysphonia can be assured.

Sarah is an example of a middle-aged Type 2 dysphonic. Psychological interview revealed a complex childhood history. Sarah presented with depression and anxiety symptoms. Following symptomatic voice therapy she was referred to psychology for CBT. In particular, treatment focused around her difficulties with expression of feelings, low self-esteem, anxiety symptoms.

For the full case history see Chapter 10, pp. 181–5.

SUMMARY

- Symptomatic voice therapy techniques are essential to the successful management of psychogenic voice disorders and most frequently are used early on in the treatment process.
- The initial approach taken by the therapist will depend largely on whether the patient presents with aphonia or dysphonia.
- Restoration of voice using symptomatic voice therapy techniques should be the primary goal of the initial session with the aphonic patient.
- Type 1 (classical hysterical) aphonics are unlikely to benefit from voice therapy techniques. Strong resistance and detachment from the aphonic during symptomatic voice therapy attempts to restore voice may be important diagnostic indicators of this group.
- Type 1 patients should be referred on to psychiatry.
- Type 3 (psychogenic-habituated) aphonics are likely to achieve total or near total resolution of symptoms using voice therapy techniques alone.

- Type 3 dysphonic patients will benefit from symptomatic voice therapy techniques and the likelihood of recurrence of their symptoms may be minimised by raised awareness of stress management techniques and a raised awareness of the association between stress, conflicts and vocal tension.
- Type 2 (cognitive behavioural) aphonics may achieve resolution of their symptoms rapidly using voice therapy techniques but require a combined CBT approach to sustain vocal improvements. A minority require CBT before voice therapy can become effective.
- Type 2 dysphonic patients will benefit most from a combined CBT and voice therapy approach that follows on from a comprehensive assessment.
- Therapeutic style and the type of verbal feedback given is of paramount importance when working with the aphonic.
- **Dysphonic** patients may require a more gradual approach to voice restoration than the aphonic and tend to be more complex.

6 Assessing Anxiety in Voice Patients

In the first part of this chapter we will present a model of anxiety reactions as viewed from a CBT perspective. This will be followed by a description of how to assess symptoms of anxiety and how to help your patient gather the data you will need to carry out a comprehensive formulation and intervention.

UNDERSTANDING ANXIETY

The foundation of anxiety is in a biological, inherited or innate reaction to threat or danger. The subjective, emotional response of feeling anxiety is only one element in a complex set of reactions. Together, these responses alert individuals to the presence of danger and prepare them for defensive, self-protective action. Thus, anxiety can be seen as an emotional alarm bell that sounds when threat is perceived. The alarm bell makes the individual more awake or alert and ready to ward off or run from dangers. This is why an intense anxiety reaction is referred to as a fight-or-flight response and why the universal theme underlying all anxiety conditions is the theme of threat or feeling threatened. This can be illustrated by the following examples from different developmental stages:

- Bad parenting will make an infant feel threatened and vulnerable because basic physical and emotional needs are not being met with any consistency.
- An older child may have difficulty with school work and be afraid of criticism from his or her teacher and parents.
- A teenager may develop acne and fear the ridicule of peers.
- A young man in his twenties may be anxious about losing his job and becoming financially insecure.
- A middle-aged woman may feel threatened by seeing her husband talking to another woman.
- An elderly man may have physical symptoms which make him believe his life is in danger from heart disease.

These examples illustrate how anxiety can be experienced at any stage in the life cycle and can result from feeling threatened emotionally or psychologically (e.g. developing acne or losing a partner) or from a genuine physical danger (e.g. having symptoms that might be life threatening).

BIOLOGICAL CHANGES ASSOCIATED WITH PERCEIVED THREAT

The perception of threat usually triggers the following changes as part of the physical preparation to fight or flee: increase in pupil dilation, muscular tension, brain wave activity, breathing, heart rate, oxygen consumption, adrenaline and lactate levels in the blood, blood pressure, peristalsis, and perspiration. At the same time, it decreases the flow of saliva, galvanic skin resistance and disrupts various biochemical functions, which help us fight off infection.

BEHAVIOURAL CHANGES ASSOCIATED WITH PERCEIVED THREAT

The perception of threat can be seen in observable behavioural changes such as rigid, defensive posture and muscular tension (such as raised shoulders or clenched fists); restlessness or agitation; physically moving away from, or phobic avoidance of, the perceived source of threat; and rapid breathing or hyperventilation.

Psychologically, the perception of threat triggers cognitive *and* emotional changes including changes in thoughts and images, as well as feelings that can be graded from nervousness, anxiety, fear, panic, and terror. Thoughts may become speeded up and images may be particularly vivid or detailed or the person may have difficulty concentrating, ordering or collecting their thoughts.

A UNIFIED AND UNIVERSAL REACTION TO PERCEIVED THREAT

These physical, behavioural, cognitive and emotional changes all play a part in the survival of threat. For example, if the danger is a physical threat then, visually, we have to see clearly what we are dealing with. Hence, the pupils dilate. If we are going to act quickly we must be alert. Hence, the release of adrenaline, the emotional stimulus of anxiety or fear, and the rapid processing of information in vivid thoughts and images. If we are going to fight or run, muscle tone must be increased. Hence, muscular skeletal muscles become tense. To fight or run, we also need to have instant access to energy. Hence, the release of sugar into the blood stream. In order to burn up the energy, we need more oxygen. Hence, we breathe more rapidly.

The same psychophysical reactions occur when facing forms of psychological or non-physical threat. A good example is the common experience of stage fright where the threat is purely psychological: fear of forgetting your lines, fear of failing in front of a large number of people, fear of being judged or criticised by others, fear of embarrassment and loss of self-esteem. Although there is no physical threat, the person reacts as though his or her life was in real danger and this triggers the same physical and emotional responses.

PSYCHOLOGICAL CHANGES ASSOCIATED WITH PERCEIVED THREAT

It should also be noted that if these physical changes are occurring regularly or even constantly over a period they are likely to take a toll on the body. For example, frequent stress may have the effect of one feeling continually at the starting gate, poised to go.

For some people the physiological reactions focus on the larynx so that vocal folds adduct, extrinsic laryngeal muscles contract and breathing rate increases.

HOW THOUGHTS AND IMAGES INCREASE ANXIETY

Shakespeare wrote: 'nothing is good or bad but thinking makes it so'. He was probably paraphrasing a statement made by the Stoic philosopher Epictatus: 'Men are not worried by things, but by their ideas about things. When we meet with difficulties, become anxious or troubled, let us not blame others, but rather ourselves, that is, our ideas about things.' (This translation cited by Powell 2000).

The way in which thought can create and increases anxiety can be illustrated by the following case example. A taxi driver suddenly feels light-headed while ferrying a customer. He has a history of depression and anxiety dating back to the sudden death of his father from a heart attack ten years earlier. Just over a year ago he had chest pains and breathlessness following a workout in his gym and around this time a friend of the same age died suddenly. Following these events and despite medical reassurance that he is in good health, he visits his GP regularly with minor complaints, believing that his symptoms reflect something more sinister. For example, when he has a boil or suffers from diarrhoea, he remains convinced it is skin or bowel cancer despite reassurance by his doctor. In this way he is, as Epictatus suggests, 'worried by' his 'ideas about things'; an ordinary skin complaint and upset stomach are visualised as symptoms of life-threatening illness. On the occasion when he felt light-headed while driving his taxi he recalls previous times when this feeling has preceded a panic attack. He has thoughts about being embarrassed by a panic attack in front of his passenger. The anticipation and the fear of embarrassment make him agitated and precipitate feelings of panic. Interestingly, analysis of events in the course of treatment indicate that he often feels better if he has a sugary drink and that his symptoms tend to emerge in association with long periods without eating. This suggests that low blood sugar level may precipitate feeling light-headed and that if he made his food intake more regular then his symptoms would decline. Similarly, if he reassures himself with thoughts that the light-headedness is nothing more than low blood sugar level and that it will pass if he has something to eat – rather than anticipating a distressing panic attack – he will be less likely to feel ill. Clark (1996) and Salkovskis (1996) have emphasised how easily *sensations* (e.g. dizziness) lead to *thoughts/interpretations* (e.g. 'I'm going to panic') and trigger an *emotional state* that fuels a panic reaction. This turns into a vicious cycle as the panic symptoms can produce sensations that fuel a further stream of fearful thoughts.

Another example might be that a voice patient is offered reassurance by the consultant that her symptoms are not serious, but she still suspects she has symptoms of throat cancer. Her anxious state of mind makes it more difficult for her to relax and to benefit from her voice exercises. The anxiety and worry also makes her immune system less robust and she contracts several throat infections, not only affecting her voice and giving her a sore throat but reinforcing her belief that there is something physically wrong that is not going to get better.

Thus, a major part of treating anxiety disorders is to assess in detail the way that events trigger specific sorts of thoughts that feed anxiety reactions or push normal arousal levels to unnecessary extremes.

A PANIC ATTACK

The term **panic attack** is commonly used to describe the physical, psychological, emotional symptoms that accompany an intense surge of anxiety. Most sufferers are greatly reassured and helped by the therapist explaining the symptoms as outlined above. Using terms to describe what is happening such as 'a response to threat'; 'feeling threatened physically and psychologically'; 'alerting oneself to danger'; 'the fight-or-flight response'; and explaining what symptoms are and why they are there, and how thoughts and images help or hinder, can be very helpful to someone trying to make sense of their experience. Because sufferers instinctively leave or avoid situations that they associate with panic, using safety behaviours in order to feel better and reinforcing the belief that this is the only thing that helps, the most helpful treatment is behavioural exposure in which the patient is encouraged to ride out the attack until symptoms decline, thus demonstrating that the feared consequence such as fainting, dying, becoming a laughing stock, does not occur.

AVOIDANCE BEHAVIOUR

Avoidance of things which cause unpleasant feelings is something everyone experiences in day-to-day life, whether this is as mundane as a child putting off a boring task like doing homework or as an adult completing a tax return, or whether this involves something more profound emotionally, which would include situations causing anxiety, physical discomfort, and/or pain.

Since animals are largely motivated by the pleasure principle, they have a strong tendency to avoid whatever is unpleasant or unrewarding and to seek out pleasant or rewarding experiences. Since anxiety is a feeling most people find unrewarding, it is usual that situations that trigger anxiety will also foster avoidance behaviour. In turn, since this avoidance causes the anxiety to decline, the avoidance is immediately rewarded or reinforced by positive feelings.

Situations that require assertive behaviour commonly cause anxiety in people. A person can usually avoid the anxiety by being unassertive. Since the increased anxiety associated with being assertive is avoided, the avoidance is rewarded (because avoidance reduces the anxiety) and this reinforces passive behaviour. A person with this pattern of behaviour has to learn ways of controlling the anxiety that makes them avoid assertiveness and probably needs to practise these skills in order to become proficient, starting with situations that are not too threatening. This is often important when considering the treatment of PVD where the fear of assertiveness and fear of expressing feelings inhibit voice production. PVD patients need help in overcoming their anxiety and avoidance behaviour and in learning to assert themselves.

Because of the role avoidance plays in anxiety disorders, the therapist needs to be able to recognise the operation of this behavioural response and the fact that it is self-reinforcing in a way which shapes and cements maladaptive patterns of behaviour. Fortunately, a number of methods can be used to alter even highly entrenched avoidance habits.

ASSESSING ANXIETY

The frequent presence of musculoskeletal tension, interpersonal relationship difficulties, conflicts over assertiveness and self-expression, feeling burdened by family responsibilities and the sense of powerlessness in patients with psychogenic voice disorder, suggest that anxiety is undoubtedly an important feature in this condition. The therapist will want to make a detailed assessment of the causes of anxiety by using interviewing skills, questionnaires and daily record sheets, before considering their treatment strategies.

INTERVIEWING SKILLS

When attempting to gain information from a client it will be important to look out for factors that may have predisposed the person to anxiety. This might include assessing exposure in life to such things as early separation experiences from care givers, poor bonding to care givers, disrupted parenting, family difficulties (rows, drink or drug problems, physical and sexual abuse, etc.), parental separations, fostering, multiple changes of school, bullying, educational difficulties, difficult adolescence, socialising problems, bereavements, major life traumas, and various adult relationship problems. These areas should be covered in the course of history taking and placed in the context of the recent life events that have propelled the patient into treatment.

QUESTIONNAIRES

A number of questionnaires have been developed to assess anxiety. The voice therapist will find these easy to administer and score. Probably the best known amongst speech and language therapists is the Irritability – Depression – Anxiety Scale (IDAS) (Snaith et al. 1978). Alternatively, the Hospital Anxiety and Depression Scale (HADS) (Zigmond and Snaith 1983) can be used as a quick screening device. Powell (2000) has published a version of this scale and this is reproduced on p. 110 as Table 6.1. The Beck and Steer (1990) Beck Anxiety Inventory can be recommended for quickly covering common symptomatology and because it provides a guide to severity. The Physical Symptoms Inventory, Table 6.2, and the Worrying Thoughts Questionnaire, Table 6.3, described by Powell (2000) can be helpful in highlighting somatic symptoms and the type of negative preoccupations associated with anxiety (see pp. 111–2). The Young Schema Questionaire (Young and Brown 2003) also elicits thoughts which feed anxiety and can compliment the Worrying Thoughts Questionnaire in providing an indication of the schemas underlying the anxiety. The Young Schema Questionnaire, scoring details, information

Table 6.1: Hospital Anxiety and Depression Scale

Please indicate how you are feeling now, or how you have been feeling in the last day or two, by ticking the column to the right of each of the following statements:

	Yes definitely	Yes sometimes	No, not much	No, not at all
1 I wake early and then sleep badly for the rest of the night.				
2 I get very frightened or have panic feelings for apparently no reason at all.				
3 I feel miserable and sad.				
4 I feel anxious when I go out of the house on my own.				
5 I have lost interest in things.				
6 I get palpitations, or a sensation of 'butterflies' in my stomach or chest.				
7 I have a good appetite.				
8 I feel scared or frightened.				
9 I feel life is not worth living.				
10 I still enjoy the things I used to.				
11 I am restless and can't keep still.				
12 I am more irritable than usual.				
13 I feel as if I have slowed down.				
14 Worrying thoughts constantly go through my mind.				

For scorer's use only:
Anxiety: (2, 4, 6, 8, 11, 12, 14)   **A**

Depression: (1, 3, 5, 7, 9, 10, 13)   **D**

Scoring–3, 2, 1, and 0 are given respectively to responses in columns 1, 2, 3 and 4, e.g. responses in the first column are all given 3; responses in the second column are given 2, and so on.

A cut off point of 8–10 is suggested on each scale as scores below or in this range do not indicate the presence of abnormal anxiety or depression.

Reproduced with permission from *The Mental Health Handbook*, Trevor Powell, Speechmark, Bicester, 2000.

Table 6.2: Physical Symptoms Inventory

Please tick the appropriate choice as to how often you have experienced the following physical symptoms during the last two weeks.

	Not at all	Occasionally	Often	Most of the time
1 Palpitations				
2 Breathlessness/rapid breathing				
3 Chest pains or discomfort				
4 Choking or smothering sensation				
5 Dizziness or feeling unsteady				
6 Tingling or numbness				
7 Hot and/or cold flushes				
8 Sweating				
9 Fainting				
10 Trembling or shaking				
11 Feeling sick				
12 Upset stomach/diarrhoea				
13 Headaches/migraine				
14 Dry mouth: difficulty swallowing				
15 Feeling of unreality				
16 Tension in jaw/neck/shoulders				
17 Jelly legs				
18 Any other physical symptoms				

Reproduced with permission from *The Mental Health Handbook*, Trevor Powell, Speechmark, Bicester, 2000.

Table 6.3: Worrying Thought Questionnaire

This section deals with your thoughts and worries about your anxiety. Please tick the appropriate choice as to how often you have experienced the following thoughts during the last two weeks.

	Not at all	Occasionally	Often	Most of the time
1 I'm going to have a heart attack.				
2 I'm going to faint.				
3 I'm going to look a fool.				
4 Things are getting worse and worse.				
5 People are looking at me.				
6 I'm going to go mad.				
7 I'm going to be too anxious to speak properly.				
8 I'm not going to be able to cope.				
9 I'm going to have a panic attack.				
10 There is something physically wrong with me. I'm ill.				
11 Why do other people cope better than I do?				
12 I can't face up to this because I will not be able to do it.				
13 I'm under a great deal of stress at the moment.				
14 Any other worrying thoughts.				

Reproduced with permission from *The Mental Health Handbook*, Trevor Powell, Speechmark, Bicester, 2000.

about related assessment forms and an invaluable introduction to Schema Therapy can be found on *www.schematherapy.com*

Scoring

When scoring the Physical Symptoms Inventory and the Worrying Thought Questionaire, the SLT may want to score the responses in the four columns in the following way: 0, 1, 2, 3 (that is, 0 for any response in column 1; 1 for any response in column 2 and so on for columns 3 and 4). Total scores should then be a reflection of symptom severity.

SELF-OBSERVATION

Self-observation is a core skill in carrying out data collection and there are a number of ways in which the therapist encourages this.

1 When describing the CBT model the therapist highlights the importance of self-observation as a means of personal discovery, change and problem solving. Since the expression **self-observation** may not be familiar to the patient, the therapist should give examples of what is meant and can use it interchangeably with terms such as self-awareness, watchfulness, mindfulness and self-monitoring.

2 To begin with the therapist can stress the importance of observing the internal monologue or dialogue that makes up our thoughts, taking note of any thinking errors and the impact these have on emotions.

3 With this the therapist can emphasise that if the thoughts that influence our feelings and behaviour remain unobserved, we continue in the same old, habitual way and change is more difficult if not impossible.

4 The therapist can then illustrate how observation or mindfulness of negative thoughts, as well as emotions, physical states and behavioural reactions, can be used as triggers to practise alternative, positive, counteracting responses (e.g. implementing positive thoughts, physical relaxation, slowing down when rushing, etc.).

5 To practice and foster self-observation, the therapist sets homework in the form of daily record sheets and will use the review of this homework to reinforce success in self-awareness and data collection.

6 Finally, the therapist can exploit the use of cueing devices as a means of increasing the frequency of awareness and self-observation. Almost anything can be used as a cueing device. A good example can be found in Aldous Huxley's last novel, *Island* (1964). In order to be more aware and live more in the present moment, the people of Huxley's mythical utopia have trained the local mynah birds to repeat the phrase 'Here and now boy, here and now.' Usually, therapists are forced to rely on less exotic help! Fortunately, there are some simple alternatives.

Table 6.4: Daily record sheet #1

Daily Record Sheet				
Date	Situation	Level of Anxiety 0–10	Thoughts/Images	Response

Table 6.5: Daily record sheet #2

Daily Record Sheet		
Date	Situation	Anxious thoughts/reactions, etc.

Table 6.6: Daily record sheet #3

Daily Record Sheet			
Date	Situation	Negative (irrational) thought	Positive (rational) thoughts

Table 6.7: Daily record sheet #4

Please make an entry whenever you notice a definite increase in anxiety.				
Date/time	Description of situation	Anxiety level: 0–10	Description of (a) physical feelings (b) thoughts	Coping method	Anxiety level after: 0–10

Reproduced with permission from *The Mental Health Handbook*, Trevor Powell, Speechmark, Bicester, 2000.

If a patient has a watch with a bleep, this can be set to sound regularly in order to cue self-observation. If the watch does not have a bleeper, the patient can place a small red sticker on its face so that the habit of checking the time will bring the sticker into view and remind the user to self-observe. If the patient does not wear a watch, the sticker can be placed on objects that are used frequently in the course of a day: shaving mirror, briefcase, car keys, purse or wallet, pen, phone, filing cabinet, lunchbox, etc. Instead of a red sticker it is also possible to use cue cards that are left in regularly frequented places such as the kitchen or office and which ask specific questions like 'what are you doing?/ thinking?/feeling?'

DAILY RECORD SHEETS

Keeping a record of *what* triggers anxiety, *how bad* the anxiety is and *when* and *where* it occurs is essential. (See Tables 6.4, 6.5, 6.6 and 6.7 pp. 114–7.) Therapists wishing to make a detailed analysis of the patient's anxiety problem should ask the patient to keep a daily record which – depending on the information required – covers the following:

- situation or event triggering anxiety
- degree of anxiety
- thoughts/images and physical feelings associated with anxiety
- response to anxiety

There are various ways in which to collect this information and the therapist may need to design forms for individual needs but Table 6.7 is an example of how most of these questions could be covered on one form.

Using an appropriate daily record sheet will enable the therapist to make a more detailed assessment of the factors in the client's life that trigger anxiety. They are designed to highlight the cognitive, emotional and behavioural reactions to these events. For many clients it can be easier starting with a simple two-column form. The form can be made more complex as the person learns to challenge negative cognitions and replace them with positive thoughts (see Tables 6.5, 6.6 and 6.7).

SUMMARY

- This chapter has introduced the reader to a model of anxiety that has biological, behavioural, emotional and cognitive elements, a model that stresses the important part played by perceived threat, whether physical or psychological, and how thoughts and images can increase anxiety, panic and avoidance behaviour.
- In assessing anxiety and gathering data, we have described a range of anxiety symptoms, emphasised the therapist's role in interviewing and using questionnaires, and the patient's role in applying self-observation and keeping daily record sheets.

7 Treating Anxiety in Voice Patients

In this chapter we will describe some common cognitive behavioural treatment strategies that have been developed as a means of treating anxiety. The description covers stress reduction techniques, target setting, cognitive and self-instructional training, the use of prompt cards, role-playing and exposure. Familiarity with these techniques should equip the voice therapist with a range of treatment options for each individual. Rather than having a treatment approach centred on the use of one method only, the voice therapist will draw upon several means of problem solving. Before commencing the therapy, however, it is important to give the patient an explanation concerning the rationale behind your treatment approach.

EXPLAINING THE TREATMENT RATIONALE

Giving an explanation as to the model of anxiety and its treatment is important. The patient should be given a clear explanation at the end of the first or early assessment sessions as to how the therapist pictures the problems and why certain treatment strategies would be appropriate.

1 Provide a description of the fight-or-flight response illustrated by examples of feeling physically and emotionally threatened. Two examples that serve this purpose well are (i) suddenly encountering a charging bull and (ii) without fore-warning, being asked to make a public speech on a subject about which you know very little. Get the patient to describe how they might feel if confronted with a situation of this sort and, when going into these examples, make sure you include descriptions of both psychological and physical changes, such as changes in thoughts and feelings and heart and breathing rates.

2 Provide a description of the way major physical and psychosocial processes interact with one another. The description should be in a simple language but convey concepts related to the influence of biological predisposition and developmental life experiences on cognitions, emotions, biophysical states and behaviour. In practice, this may not be as difficult as it may first appear. The following is just one way a therapist might attempt to convey information about the model, its focus and style of treatment:

'Getting anxious is a common experience but some people may have a predisposition to become more anxious than others. Children vary a great deal in temperament. Some children are nervous and clinging in new situations, some are quite the opposite. However, even a confident and independent child gets anxious at times, and different experiences as children develop might influence their tendency to become anxious.

For example, if children have a lot of experiences that make them feel insecure they may be more prone to anxiety symptoms. Similarly, major stress in later life can produce anxiety reactions in almost everyone. Given enough stress, most people will feel anxious and panicky.'

'Most of us think of anxiety simply as an emotion, but it has other features as well. For example, while the emotion of anxiety might arise out of social situations or relationships (e.g., a conflict with your husband), it is also influenced by your thoughts about these events (e.g., believing that you will never be able to express your views or that he will leave you if you do so), and these can make your feelings worse. Emotions of anxiety also have a physical quality (e.g., palpitations, hyperventilation, musculoskeletal tension, sweating, churning stomach, loss of appetite, weak legs, etc.) and a psychological element in the sense that it causes problems with attention, concentration and thinking things through clearly. Finally, the emotion of anxiety also affects our behaviour. For example, because most of us avoid things that feel unpleasant, we will find ourselves automatically avoiding situations or challenges that provoke anxiety.'

'In trying to help someone overcome an anxiety problem, it is usually important to look at the different facets of anxiety in order to consider what strategies might be helpful in bringing about change. For example, the physical symptoms of musculoskeletal tension might be treated with progressive muscular relaxation and rapid relaxation; the negative thoughts that feed this tension might be changed through cognitive therapy techniques; while a stressful relationship that has caused the anxiety and the avoidance behaviour which has maintained it might be altered by setting graded targets to practise assertiveness. Thus, in therapy, time is usually spent looking at the different forms anxiety takes, trying to understand what causes and maintains it, and then trying a combination of appropriate, practical strategies to shift the problem or help you tolerate the symptoms better.'

The above example is obviously idealised in the sense that few of us explain what we are doing as succinctly as this but it is important in CBT to take every opportunity to provide our patients with a treatment rationale.

PROGRESSIVE MUSCULAR RELAXATION

Systematically stretching or tensing and relaxing the major muscles of the body as a means of inducing mental tranquillity is an ancient technique, e.g., the yoga asanas. However, a relaxation method, initially developed and researched by Jacobson (1938), known as Progressive Muscular Relaxation (PMR) has been the most widely used by psychologists. Training in PMR can be seen as a means of teaching anxious individuals a coping strategy which, in combination with other CBT techniques, will help them face situations they would normally avoid. In its original form PMR can be quite time consuming but patients report benefiting from shorter versions that can take less than 15 minutes. Brevity can be valuable because it makes it quicker to learn, it is easier to fit into busy daily routines, and it reduces 'practice fatigue' or the boredom that lowers motivation to keep practising the technique. The following describes the progressive muscular relaxation we have been using and how this forms the basis for developing other skills within a stress reduction programme

THE INTRODUCTION

Initially the therapist should give information about autonomic arousal and muscular tension in order to provide a rationale for focus. Emphasis should be placed on re-discovering the neglected skills of relaxing and breaking the bad habit of being tense. Since individuals occasionally have a negative reaction to relaxation, this should be mentioned, suggesting that unfamiliarity with being relaxed or the surfacing of suppressed emotions may, in rare cases, cause anxious feelings. Explaining that feeling anxious is rare, usually only fleeting and not a precursor of something worse, will normally reassure the person.

THE PROCEDURE

The patient needs to sit or lie comfortably – with closed eyes to help concentration – and should practise the exercises at a time when, or in a place where, they will not be inter-rupted. In some cases there may be physical reasons (e.g., back injury) for doing an exercise particularly gently or omitting it altogether. Throughout the series of exercises the patient is instructed to be aware of the sensation being experienced and to note the contrasts in feeling between tension and relaxation. The 12 steps of an abbreviated vers-ion of PMR outlined in Butcher, Elias and Raven (1993) are cited in full below as a guide:

1   Clenching the hands into tight fists, holding this for a moment while being aware of this sensation and then releasing the tension. Repeat.
2   Clenching hands into fists, bringing fists up to the shoulders so that arms are bent and tense throughout, holding for a moment, then releasing the tension by slowly dropping the arms and uncurling the fingers. Repeat.
3   Wrinkling the forehead into a worried frown, holding a moment before allowing the brow to relax and become 'smooth and soft'. Repeat.
4   Screwing up the eyes by pressing down with the eyelids. Releasing the tension. Repeat.
5   Tensing the lower half of the face by pressing lips together tightly. Releasing the tension. Repeat.
6   Turning the head slowly as far to the right as possible, holding a moment, then turning it slowly around as far to the left as possible, holding a moment, bringing the head back to the centre, then slowly lowering it forward so that the chin presses into the chest and the muscles can be felt stretching along the back of the neck, holding a moment before returning the head to a normal, relaxed, upright position.
7   Lifting the shoulders as high as possible, being sure not to tense the arms in order to assist this but to keep them limp and relaxed. (When the shoulders have relaxed, ask if clients can drop their shoulders even further.) Repeat.

8   Arching or bowing the back by gently pushing forward with the stomach and back with the shoulders, then releasing the tension. Repeat.

9   Taking a slow, deep diaphragmatic breath by filling up with air low into the lungs, rather than the chest, and after holding a moment, releasing the breath as slowly as possible. Repeat.

10   Tensing or knotting the stomach, then releasing the tension. Repeat.

11   Tensing the legs by (a) pushing downward with the heels, holding a moment and relaxing, (b) pushing down with the toes, holding a moment and relaxing, (c) stretching the toes and feet upward or backward towards the shins, holding and relaxing.

12   When these exercises have been completed, clients are asked to go back over each group of muscles in order to see if they are still relaxed or whether any tension has returned. The instructions are as follows:

Feel the relaxation in your hands and fingers; your wrists; the forearms and upper arms. See if you can relax even further. If there is any tension just let go of it ... Feel the relaxation in your forehead; round the eyes and eyelids; your cheeks and lips and jaw. If you feel any tension just let go of it ... Feel the relaxation around your neck and deep down in your shoulders and shoulder blades. See if you can drop your shoulders even further ... Feel the relaxation in your lower back; in the slow rhythm of your breathing; in your stomach; and then feel the relaxation spreading down from your body into your legs; your thighs; calves; ankles; feet; and right to the tip of your toes ... You should now be completely relaxed ... Notice how pleasant relaxation feels and how it contrasts with the sensation of tension ... Just enjoy the relaxation for a few moments ... Now, slowly rouse yourself up to go about your every day activities. Try not to lose this sense of deep muscular relaxation. Watch out for tension returning. If you notice an increase in muscular tension, just practise letting go of it and see if you can recapture the sensation of deep relaxation.

RAPID STRESS CONTROL

Once patients have learned PMR they can begin to learn more sophisticated stress reduction techniques. These can be employed whenever the person needs coping strategies in a stressful or challenging situation. The method of rapid stress control described by Butcher Elias and Raven (1993) involves four procedures that form the basis of a simple self-help programme: (1) self-observation, (2) positive self-instruction, (3) slow diaphragmatic breathing and (4) rapid relaxation. The procedure has been produced on audio-cassette tape with a self-help booklet (Butcher 2000).

SELF-OBSERVATION

As described earlier, self-observation involves becoming aware of the physical and psychological features of anxiety, in particular, getting into the good habit of regularly checking for signs of muscular tension and whether this is connected with negative thoughts. The idea is that regular use of self-observation and stress control strategies will inhibit the build-up of tension. The practice of self-observation is not only encouraged but is stimulated through the use of a cueing device in the form of a small red dot stuck on the face of the person's watch or any place they might look frequently, such as a mirror or telephone.

THOUGHT CATCHING AND POSITIVE SELF-INSTRUCTION

If self-observation reveals the presence of negative thoughts, the person is asked to question the validity and necessity of these thoughts and to find positive alternatives. The analysis of negative automatic thoughts might be as thorough and systematic as the steps outlined later on page 126 where the person asks: 'What is the evidence for thinking this way?' 'What alternative views are there?' 'What is the effect of thinking the way I do?' 'What sort of thinking error am I making?' and 'What action can I take?' Alternatively, the person can look for the self-statements that contain imperative or overgeneralised beliefs like 'should', 'must', 'ought', 'never' and 'can't' which feed anxiety (see Dryden & Ellis 1988). These can then be changed to more positive and self-supportive statements. For example, when preparing to speak her mind to a dominating partner a person notices the thoughts: 'I must get this right but I'm too nervous and I'll make mistakes. I can't stand making mistakes and hearing his critical comments.' She catches the thoughts and uses thought challenging or positive self-instruction: 'I don't have to do it perfectly, only as well as I can. It's OK to be nervous. Besides, I'm only nervous because I am worrying about him being critical. If I stop worrying about that, it follows that I won't be nervous. Anyway, what's the big deal about getting it wrong? Everyone makes mistakes. Who says I can't cope with criticism. He might not agree with my views but I have a right to hold them. I'm acting as though getting it wrong or being criticised would kill me. If it goes wrong I might feel a bit wound up but I'll recover. Anyhow, I don't *know* anything bad will happen. I'll do my best and use it as a chance to practise keeping relaxed under pressure.'

The patient should also be encouraged to get into a self-instruction habit of simply saying, 'relax', so that this becomes a cue to the following relaxation exercises.

SLOW, DIAPHRAGMATIC BREATHING

Anxiety has a physical effect on how we breathe and creates a pattern of breathing that is rapid and shallow. This hyperventilation is part of the preparation for action and occurs because fight or flight requires a speedy intake of fresh oxygen and the expulsion of CO_2. When rapid thoracic breathing occurs without action, oxygen and carbon dioxide levels in the blood become unbalanced and cause symptoms of light-headedness, remoteness, dizziness, and numbness or pins and needles in the hands and fingers. Slow breathing using the diaphragm is a way of inhibiting hyperventilation and its unpleasant side effects. When practised, many people find it has the psychological effect of making them feel more calm and grounded.

In breathing slowly with the diaphragm the person focuses on (1) slowing down the breathing and (2) filling up the lower lungs, rather than the chest. This can be demonstrated to the patient by placing one hand on your own chest and the other where your stomach joins the arch of the ribcage. As you breathe in, the hand on your stomach should move significantly more than the hand on your chest.

On observing a tendency to breathe with the chest or as part of the following self-instruction to relax and carry out rapid stress control, the individual should take a slow diaphragmatic breath, hold it for a moment or two and release the air as slowly as possible, repeating until the breathing becomes more tranquil. Focusing on breathing out *as slowly as possible* after taking a diaphragmatic breath helps re-balance the oxygen and CO_2 levels in the blood and reduces the possibility of light-headedness.

RAPID RELAXATION

As the person slows down breathing he or she also focuses on relaxing physically. An ideal way to carry this out is simply to relax individual muscles as described earlier in Step 12 of Progressive Muscular Relaxation (p. 120). The person focuses on relaxing their hands, wrists, arms, forehead, eyes, cheeks, lips, jaw, neck, shoulders, shoulder blades, lower back, chest, stomach, thighs, calves and feet. Because the practitioner should be familiar with Step 12 from practising Progressive Muscular Relaxation, he or she will find this an easy procedure to follow. However, it may take some practice before they can use the technique to fully relax in a challenging situation. Best results are gained from *frequent practice* and *early application of the technique* before physical tension builds up.

ACCEPTANCE

Recent developments in behavioural and cognitive therapy (for example, Hayes et al. 2003; Segal et al. 2002) have indicated that individuals suffering from anxiety and depression do better in treatment if, instead of *trying to control their emotions*, they change their focus to *accepting the discomfort* that comes with these feelings. In fact, research has shown that efforts to control emotional states tend to make the emotions intensify. Furthermore, when the therapy includes a key emphasis on abandoning efforts at emotional regulation and focuses on accepting feelings without resisting them, outcome studies show participants do at least as well, and in some ways better, than in standard CBT (see Eifert & Forsyth 2005, for an elaboration of this important emphasis in treatment). Hence, it is very important that the therapist makes it clear to their patient at the start of treatment that any coping or stress reduction strategies have limited value and may inadvertently make things worse if all their effort is focused on emotional regulation. In other words, the patient should be informed that while coping strategies may have a place (for example, learning to question unhelpful or negative thoughts when feeling uncomfortable about expressing views), these strategies will be of limited value, at best only an adjunct or peripheral to the core skill of accepting the discomfort that comes with facing something emotionally disturbing, not putting effort into controlling emotions and being willing to accept, tolerate or 'hold' discomfort in order to move in a valued direction. (For a comprehensive description of this emphasis in therapy, see Hayes et al. 2003.)

TARGET SETTING

Cognitive behavioural treatment sessions are usually concluded with target setting. The type of targets set in treating anxiety disorders might typically include such things as:

- daily practise of Progressive Muscular Relaxation
- daily practise of rapid stress reduction techniques
- practise of other activities that might be relaxing (e.g., listening to music, reading, yoga, exercise, meditation)
- graded practise of behaviours that are usually avoided or dropping safety behaviours (e.g., speaking your mind, phoning a friend).

COGNITIVE RETRAINING

The thoughts of most people, as Albert Ellis has highlighted, are often dominated by various types of thinking errors, particularly the imperatives *should*, *must*, and *ought*, which make them feel anxious and, at most times, can be considered unnecessary statements to oneself (Dryden & Ellis 1988). First of all, as an example, thinking, '*I must* be liked by everyone I meet' is obviously asking the impossible. (This can be challenged in therapy with '*How can I demand everyone like me? Does anybody like everyone they meet?*') Second, it is making a generalisation error. (Here a challenge might be '*Surely it's enough to be liked by some people some of the time?*') Third, by simply accepting the initial thought, the person fails to consider more deeply why this imperative to be liked might be necessary or why it seems so important. (The person can ask in response, 'Do I think it is something I must have to make me a better person or to feel okay about myself and, if so, why should I think this?')

Once patients become skilled in self-observation they should become more aware of thinking errors and begin trying out new ways of thinking. Using daily record sheets as part of cognitive retraining can be an invaluable means of gathering information and developing positive alternatives to negative thoughts. One of the easiest, most natural ways of working during the first phase of therapy is to go through the patient's record of situations producing anxious thoughts and, together, consider possible alternative ways of thinking about the situation. Once patients begin keeping their own record of attempts at using positive thoughts in anxious situations, time can be spent seeing if there are any other helpful thoughts that might be included.

Many of the dysfunctional thoughts that cause depressive feelings also provoke anxiety. Therefore, the therapist should be familiar with these types of thinking error (see pp. 140–1, 146, 149 and 151–2). However, as a framework, Beck and Emery (1985) suggest three approaches that can be particularly important in helping anxious individuals observe and challenge their cognitions. These involve getting the patient to ask: 'What is the evidence?' or 'What's another way of looking at it?' or 'So what if it happens?'

WHAT IS THE EVIDENCE?

Patients are encouraged to look for faulty logic in their thinking. For example, if patients believe everyone will think them fools if they stumble over words in a public meeting, they can explore this and will discover that (a) it is an *overgeneralisation* (people do not *always* think a person is a fool for making errors under stress and *everyone* will not think the same thought), (b) it is a *mind reading error* (you are not a mind reader and, therefore, you don't know that people are thinking badly of you) and (c) a *fortune teller error* (no-one can predict the future and just because you've thought it doesn't mean it will come true). Beck and Emery (1985) recommend using the three-column technique (a daily record sheet with three columns headed Situation, Automatic Thought and Error) so that the therapist can go through the form with patients to analyse what situations trigger automatic errors in thinking. With this they suggest it will often be helpful and necessary to provide information (e.g. when patients think their symptoms are signs of going mad, the therapist explains that the symptoms are just normal signs of anxiety). They suggest that in setting homework the therapist also encourages patients to involve themselves in hypothesis testing, that is, testing out whether or not their beliefs or the hypotheses they have about what will happen are correct (e.g. someone who believes that people will be angry if they speak their mind, will be set the target of finding ways to test whether or not this belief is true). Finally, they note that the hypothesis testing can also be carried out in the session (e.g. in the case of someone with dysphonia who says they are too anxious to ever express certain feelings, they could prove that this is not the case through role-play and practice with the therapist).

WHAT'S ANOTHER WAY OF LOOKING AT IT?

The therapeutic challenge is to generate alternative interpretations, helping the person to stand back and look at themselves or the situation more objectively or like an observer who is not emotionally involved and then helping them enlarge their perspective through generating alternative hypotheses or more realistic, accurate statements about themselves or their situation.

SO WHAT IF IT HAPPENS?

The emphasis here is assessing whether the consequences that are feared are as bad as predicted or *completely* bad. The patient can also be encouraged to develop detailed coping strategies. Beck and Emery (1985) suggest a technique they call **point/counterpoint** that can be valuable in this context. They illustrate this technique as follows:

> **Therapist:** You seem to have a lot of reasons why you believe the feared event is going to happen, why it is so terrible, and why you wouldn't be able to handle it. Since you have those arguments down so well, let's work together to dispute them with other possibilities. I'll give you the fearful ideas, and you give me the counter ideas. When you run out of positive counterpoints, we'll switch roles and I'll give the counterpoints.
>
> Beck & Emery 1985, p.208

As Beck and Emery point out, the therapist and patient continue to exchange roles and help each other to improve a counter argument. They emphasise that the therapist should present the counterpoint strongly and confidently and they highlight that the strategy generally covers four areas: '(1) the probability of the feared event; (2) its degree of awfulness; (3) the patient's ability to prevent it from occurring; and (4) the patient's ability to accept and deal with the worst possible outcome' (1985, p. 209).

The sort of thinking errors that may also be relevant in working with anxiety disorders can be found in the Schema Questionnaire. The following selection are just a few examples: *'I worry that people I feel close to will leave me or abandon me.' 'I become upset when someone leaves me alone, even for a short period of time.' 'I feel that people would take advantage of me.' 'I feel that I cannot let my guard down in the presence of other people, or else they will intensely hurt me.' 'If someone acts nicely towards me, I assume that he/she must be after something.' 'If I disappeared tomorrow, no one would notice.' 'No man/woman I desire could love me once he/she saw my defects.' 'It is my fault that my parent(s) could not love me enough.' 'I'm dull and boring in social situations.' 'I'm a failure.' 'I need other people to help me get by.' 'I'm inept in most areas of life.' 'My judgement cannot be relied upon in everyday situations.' 'I can't seem to escape the feeling that something bad is about to happen.' 'I worry a lot about pleasing other people so that they won't reject me.' 'I must be the best at most of what I do; I can't accept second best.' 'Almost nothing I do is quite good enough; I can always do better.' 'I get very irritated when people won't do what I ask them.'* The therapist searches out the thinking error in these beliefs through questions and discussion, first helping the patients challenge their assumptions, then helping them replace the beliefs with more accurate and positive self-statements.

MEICHENBAUM'S SELF-INSTRUCTIONAL TRAINING

Meichenbaum and Genest (1982) point out that self-instructional training grew from the view that the development of speech in children provides a means of initiating and inhibiting behaviour. Initially, young infants are controlled or directed by the speech of adults and older children. Later, as they develop they can be overheard giving themselves instructions or self-commands, speaking in the third person. Eventually, 'the child's covert or inner speech comes to assume a self-governing role' (p. 391). In other words, what we say to ourselves sub-vocally initiates or inhibits action. In cases of poor impulse control and anxiety, it is assumed that people have not learned to say the right things to themselves to inhibit being distracted or aggressive and to reduce or control anxiety.

Initial research with self-instructional training was with impulsive children and involved an adult performing a task while voicing out loud the positive thoughts (cognitive modelling) that the child needed to acquire in the situation. This cognitive modelling is followed by asking the child to perform the activity under the guidance of adult direction and, later, the child practises the task while giving self-instruction out loud. Next the child whispers self-instruction and, finally, performs the activity giving self-instruction sub-vocally (see Meichenbaum & Genest 1982). For example, the child with poor concentration or impulsive or aggressive behaviour, will be taken through the stages of the task at hand and helped to develop appropriate self-statements to define the problem and focus attention (e.g. 'Now what do I have to do?' 'This should be the best way' 'Don't gaze out of the window, concentrate', etc.), develop self-reinforcement or self-praise statements and, finally, helped to develop self-evaluation statements about skill and ability to correct errors, etc. In a similar way, the principles of self-instruction can be applied to adult anxiety problems where negative thoughts and anxiety interfere with concentration and reduce personal performance. Meichenbaum and Genest (1982) provide a helpful list of self-statements that can be rehearsed with the client as part of stress management or stress inoculation training:

EXAMPLES OF COPING SELF-STATEMENTS

Preparing for a stressor

What is it you have to do?
You can develop a plan to deal with it.
Just think about what you can do about it.
That's better than getting anxious.
No negative self-statements: just think rationally.
Don't worry; worry won't help anything.
Maybe what you think is anxiety is eagerness to confront the stressor.

Confronting and handling a stressor

Just psych yourself up – you can meet this challenge.
Reason your fear away.
One step at a time; you can handle the situation.
Don't think about fear, just think about what you have to do. Stay relevant.
This anxiety is what the doctor said you would feel.
It's a reminder to use your coping exercises.
This tenseness can be an ally; a cue to cope.

Relax; you're in control. Take a slow deep breath.
Ah, good.

Coping with the feeling of being overwhelmed

When fear comes, just pause.
Keep the focus on the present; what is it you have to do?
Label your fear from 0 to 10 and watch it change.
You should expect your fear to rise.
Manageable.

Reinforcing self-statements

It worked; you did it.
Wait until you tell your therapist (or group) about this.
It wasn't as bad as you expected.
You made more out of your fear than it was worth.
Your damn ideas – that's the problem.
When you control them, you control your fear.
It's getting better each time you use the procedures.
You can be pleased with the progress you're making.
You did it!

As can be seen by some of these self-statements, there is a tendency at times for the therapist to focus on thoughts about emotional regulation (e.g. 'Relax; you're in control') which (as discussed earlier, p. 124), may be counterproductive, but otherwise many self-statements are used to encourage the patient to view the anxiety in a positive way (e.g. 'This anxiety is what the doctor said you would feel;' 'You should expect your fear to rise'), to accept it and not struggle to control or reject it.

PROMPT CARDS

Prompt cards are often used as part of cognitive retraining. These are usually developed from issues that come up in therapy and where the patient needs a way of establishing a habit of thinking along helpful lines in certain situations. The patient carries the card on their person in order to refer to it whenever necessary. The following case examples illustrate how patients might use prompt cards.

Prompt cards were used to help a patient whose anxiety related to the core fear of not being able to look after herself in her day-to-day life. This fear so dominated her thinking that she felt herself to be vulnerable and needy of help despite strong evidence to the contrary; she was, in fact, quite successful in managing her personal and professional life. (Many of her fears could be traced back to her poor relationship with a domineering, rigid, highly critical father who undermined her confidence in herself.) Prior to developing the prompt card the patient was asked to keep a daily record for a week in which she ticked the hours in the day when she looked after herself successfully (e.g. getting breakfast, travelling to work, dealing with the demands of her job, meeting others, etc.) The record showed that her ability to look after herself was more than 90% of the time and, therefore, far outweighed the times when she had a sense of not being able to do this. With this information, it became possible to develop a prompt card that contained positive statements she could make about her ability to look after herself (e.g. 'My daily record *proves* I look after myself extremely well. I shouldn't exaggerate how often I have problems in this area', 'It's really quite rare for me to feel I'm not coping', etc.). The patient was encouraged to take out the card and referred to it on a regular basis, in order to boost self-assurance.

The same person also found cue cards helpful in another way. Like many patients, she had difficulty retaining the insights achieved in the therapeutic hour and at the end of the sessions found it helpful to write down things she could review during the week. For example, 'People who appear to criticise me without me knowing why make me feel anxious, helpless and weak. This comes from how my father made me feel much of the time. But I do not have to feel at fault, anxious, helpless, or weak, in response to unreasonable criticism. I should ask myself the following in these situations: Am I jumping to conclusions? Am I being irrational? Am I exaggerating what happened or what was said? Is there a better way of looking at this? Is the person who appears to be critical, the one who has a problem? etc.'

Several prompt cards were developed to help a young man whose low self-esteem and anxiety appeared to be the cause of depressive feelings and suicidal thoughts. One of the prompt cards took the form of a flow chart designed to help him see this process and all the stages in this pattern:

SELF-ESTEEM – ANXIETY – AVOIDANCE – DEPRESSION

Low self-worth → self-conscious or feeling the judgement of others → anticipatory anxiety or fear of not being able to deal with possible eventualities → avoidance → thinking I failed to deal with these in the past and present → increase in sense of low self-worth → depression.

A prompt card can be used prior to a situation in which a person has to be assertive. For example:

I have a *right* to hold these views. I have a *right* to express them. I have a *right* to ask for what I want. It is important to be straight and honest with this person. If they don't accept my view or what I request, it does not invalidate me, or my opinions. They will probably respect me for being forthright.

Prompt cards can be used in a more general way for all those situations that provoke anxiety:

> This may be a bit stressful but I've done difficult things before. So, I can do it again. I've found before that focusing my efforts on controlling anxiety doesn't really work. In fact, trying to control how I feel usually makes anxiety worse. I've learned that avoiding facing things I don't like doesn't change anything. Problems don't go away if you don't face them. It just draws out the agony. I might not like feeling anxious, but I can put up with it and I'm not going to let a little anxiety stand in the way of living my life.

Patients may also refer to cue cards when prompted by a watch-timer or by seeing a red dot stuck on the face of their watch, etc. Employing a watch-timer to prompt using a cue card was described (Butcher 1983) as part of the treatment programme for a man suffering from persistent separation anxiety with panic whenever he stopped overnight away from his house and mother. One target the patient set himself was purchasing his own place to live. However, although he found somewhere he liked, when the day came to sign contracts, he panicked and could not go through with the purchase. The thoughts precipitating the panic were that if he signed the agreement he would have to move out immediately from his current home and he would be trapped by the purchase that would be a millstone around his neck. When the patient again found an apartment he wanted to purchase, he agreed to use his watch bleeper as an hourly stimulus to read over the following self-statements that were written in the back of his pocket diary:

> 1 Even if I have taken out the mortgage, I can sell the apartment whenever I want.
> 2 Purchase of the apartment does not necessarily mean I will have to leave home immediately and it can be used for weekends only.
> 3 The apartment can be viewed simply as a wise investment and nothing more.
> 4 Relax [use the diaphragmatic breathing and physical relaxation techniques he had learned].

Although no other method of desensitisation was used, within three weeks he had reduced the frequency of the bleeper to once a day, felt only mild anxiety at the thought of the purchase, had no sleepless nights and, when the time came, completed the various arrangements and signed the legal documents without panicking.

Therapists working with psychogenic voice disorder will find that prompt cards and cueing devices such as those described above can be a helpful aid to treatment. For example, a woman with the fear of expressing her views to her husband and whose voice becomes worse at these times, might use the following prompt card when preparing to speak her mind:

1　It is important that I express myself.
2　The satisfaction of saying something will outweigh the anticipatory anxiety.
3　I don't have to say it perfectly. The important thing is saying something.
4　Even if it's not fully successful, I shouldn't exaggerate and turn a failure into a disaster. If I fail, I can still try again.
5　I don't *know* he will get angry. I can't predict the future.
6　Even if he gets angry, is that so terrible?
7　I mustn't assume he's thinking things without good evidence. I am not a mind reader.
8　It is my right to say what I think.

CREATING COGNITIVE CHANGE THROUGH ROLE-PLAYING

Role-playing not only provides an opportunity to try out new behaviours, but it is an ideal way to practise positive or helpful thinking associated with self-esteem, personal rights, and levels of performance or success. Much of this is very relevant to the anxiety experienced by people with psychogenic voice disorder. During role-playing the participants get an opportunity to (1) say things that are normally difficult for them to say, (2) get feedback on how they have performed, (3) have feedback on how it felt to hear what was said, and (4) through role reversal, actually experience how it might feel to be the other person hearing what is said.

In order to practise role-playing the therapist will need a general idea of the problem area and some details of specific problems. However, perhaps the most important skill is not only being personally uninhibited about role-playing but being able to persuade patients to lose their own performance inhibitions. The majority of practice situations are of quite short duration and do not require a great deal of acting. Most can be rehearsed while seated face-to-face. The following is an example of how role-playing might be introduced:

Therapist: So when you think about telling your husband that you would like him to help more around the house, what would you *really* like to say?
Patient: I've had it up to here with your lack of contribution!
Therapist: How do you think he'd react?
Patient: He'd get angry and start finding fault in me.
Therapist: He'd get defensive?
Patient: Yes.
Therapist: Can you think of a way of saying what you want to say that wouldn't get his back up?

Patient: He is very sensitive to criticism. I think whatever I say will make him defensive.

Therapist: What if you introduced the subject by telling him the things he's done that you've appreciated? Then he'll know you're not being *totally* critical or dismissive of him.

Patient: I'm not sure I can think of anything. He's been like this so long. He only helps out after I nag and nag him.

Therapist: So, he does help out but only if you keep on and that's what you would like to change?

Patient: Yes.

Therapist: Well, lets see how it feels to say that and to do it as though your husband was here now, as though you're speaking directly to him. Just give that a try.

Patient: OK. (After a pause.) It seems these days I'm always having to nag and nag before you help out around the house.

Therapist: Fine. OK. Now, let's look at some different ways you think your husband might respond. I can take the part of your husband and you can practise responding to my replies. That way, you can have some practice at being assertive, I can give you feedback on how you are doing or how it might feel to be in your husband's shoes. You can let me know if you think your husband might respond in some other way to what I'm doing and we can add that into the mix, and, together, we can find the strategies that work best for you and get you where you want to be. (Role-play begins.)

As highlighted in this example, the therapist draws the patient into the role-playing via the line of questioning and problem definition and by asking the patient to repeat what she said as though her husband was here now and she was speaking directly to him. Sometimes patients need a little encouragement in this but most will find they can get into the spirit of the role-playing without too much difficulty and will benefit from the rehearsal even when they feel self-conscious or that the whole thing is rather artificial. When the scene is fully analysed and rehearsed, the role-playing leads naturally to setting targets for practice in the real-life settings.

A CASE EXAMPLE OF REHEARSAL AND ROLE-PLAY WITH A COMPLEX PROBLEM

The value of role-playing as a means of preparing and rehearsing for difficult, anxiety provoking situations can be illustrated by the following case of a student, SD, who repeatedly failed his exams due to preoccupation with his emotional problems, his difficulty voicing his feelings and major communication difficulties within his family. During the build-up to one important exam SD became clinically depressed and made a serious suicidal attempt for which he was hospitalised. He described a pattern at exam times in which thoughts about his family and his own identity would crowd into his mind, causing poor concentration and poor retention of material. In illustrating the lack of communication in the family and the thoughts that preoccupied him, he described how he had discovered the birth certificate of an elder brother whose existence he had not known about. He said he was unable to ask his older sisters or his parents for more information about this. He had also discovered documents describing a court case involving a separation order because of beatings his mother received from his father. Concerning his preoccupation with his identity, SD talked of not knowing who he was, not knowing details of his family background, and of wanting to know what had happened to the members of his father's family who survived the war and migrated from Poland. Although he suspected that his father was Jewish, his father denied this.

Exploration of communication patterns within the family suggested that members avoided emotional topics and that a great deal of control was exercised through the threat of illness. For example, SD felt that his mother would not allow him to be ill because she too would become ill through worry, and because his father suffered from a heart condition SD was also careful not to cause him any stress. He expressed the view that the *combined* stresses of examinations and family tensions were behind his problem. He felt that if his family problems were sorted out he would be able to concentrate on his work and could face his exams. As he put it: 'One thing at a time, not both.'

Following his discharge from hospital, SD planned to travel home to visit his parents for four days and it was decided to focus treatment on ways of helping him (a) ask his parents the questions which preoccupied him and (b) insure that he would receive adequate answers. Basing his judgements on knowledge of his parents' previous reactions when presented with emotionally loaded topics, SD was asked to develop a scenario of conversations and events that would take place when he returned home and brought up the topic of his examination difficulties. It was planned that at the next sessions the script would be used to develop strategies that might lead to a satisfactory outcome and would form the basis of role-playing exercises.

When seen again six days later, SD had written a carefully prepared scenario. On arriving home he planned to get straight to the point, saying that he had failed his examinations and that the reason he had not done well was that the questions to do with the family intruded into his mind at examination times, would 'dart about' and make it impossible for him to function. SD imagined that his mother would reply that he was saying it was their fault for failing his exams. Originally, he wanted to say that he did blame them but, after discussion, he agreed that a reply of this sort would increase tension or conflict and cause the discussion to deteriorate into an argument. After exploring possibilities, SD agreed that the best tactic at this point was to align himself with the family by saying the following: 'I'm just as much to blame for bottling up the questions for so long. This is a problem the family share and I am only trying to overcome this for our own good, so that the family will function better.' It was also planned that he would use a similar reply if, as he predicted, his mother said he, or the subject, was making her ill. He would say, 'Yes, I can understand. It's been making me ill as well.' If, as he predicted, she attempted to leave the room, he was asked to dissuade her by stressing the importance of talking about his problem. After rehearsing these statements SD was asked to use the coming interval between therapy sessions to plan what questions he wanted to ask and how these would be phrased.

At the following meeting, two days prior to his visit home, SD brought a written list of 31 questions! These fell mainly into four areas or themes:

1 questions about his older brother
2 questions about his mother's and father's past
3 questions about documents he found describing a court case and separation order involving his parents
4 questions about relations who survived the war, who they were, what they were like, where they lived, etc.

The main emphasis of this session and in the role-playing was on alternating questions in order to begin with statements or questions that were likely to be the least threatening to his parents and suggesting and practising ways of rephrasing statements or questions so that they did not appear too attacking or lacking in empathy for his parents.

When seen following his visit home, SD reported that he was able to use a great deal of what he had rehearsed and, as a consequence, his meeting with his parents went extremely well. It had been arranged that he start asking his questions only when both parents were present. As his mother was out when he arrived home he merely greeted his father in a perfunctory way and waited in his room. On hearing his mother's return, SD joined his parents. His mother asked how he was and he replied (as planned) that he had been in hospital. His parents did not react to this, or rather, reacted as if nothing had happened, or as though it was a normal thing to mention, something which did not require comment. To break through this silence SD shouted, *'I've been in hospital!'* This forced his parents to ask what had happened.

When he replied that he could not sit his exams they immediately suggested that it must have been the pressure of work. He replied that it was not pressure in this way and explained (as rehearsed) that his difficulty was related to the family and family secrets. As predicted, his parents responded by saying that he was blaming them for his failure. As planned he replied, no, we are all to blame; a statement which calmed the situation. At this point, however, his mother said that she was feeling ill. SD took this cue and replied that the issues he wanted to discuss were making the whole family ill. His father then attempted to leave the room. This was uncharacteristic and not predicted. Rather surprisingly, his wife persuaded him to stay. At this point SD produced the birth certificate and documents he had found, and asked about his brother and the court case involving his parents.

As a result of these manoeuvres SD was told about the circumstances of his brother's birth. The elder brother was born while the parents were in Ireland at a time when the marriage was shaky and breaking up. The baby remained with his mother's parents when the couple moved to England. SD was given addresses through which he could trace his brother if he wished.

For the first time SD's father was able to talk at length and in some detail about his past and his experiences in Poland during the war. Previously, he had told SD that his grandfather had been shot by the Nazis and that he had escaped by walking to

Switzerland. He now revealed that he had seen his father tortured to death and that he had been interned in a concentration camp for the duration of the German occupation. Although deeply distressed by recounting these experiences, he was able to answer most of SD's questions. Furthermore, he was able to talk about his stormy early relationship with his wife. SD felt that his father's concentration camp experience, where he witnessed many beatings, partly explained and excused his father's violence towards his mother. His parents also gave him more information about family members who survived the war and provided him with various addresses. SD's father denied that he was Jewish and although SD continued to have suspicions about this (believing he was hiding it because it was his way of surviving the concentration camp and because his wife was a strict Irish catholic), he no longer felt that knowing one way or the other was important now that he had answers to his other questions. Towards the end of the session in which SD narrated the above he spontaneously commented that if there were an exam tomorrow, he felt confident he could sit it.

When seen after a second visit home and eight days before resitting the first two of four exams (one written and three oral examinations) he reported that the whole family was getting on better together, that his revision was going extremely well and that his rate of absorbing material was greatly improved now that his mind was not on the family issues. He said that he was confident about the examinations and he was not getting anxious because retaining information was easier. He reported some bad memories to do with his previous recent attempts at exams, which occurred mainly before sleeping; however, he was not suppressing these images and was pleased to find that as he watched them 'float past' they disappeared.

At an appointment two days before his first two examinations, SD continued to feel confident about sitting. He was using the relaxation technique he had learned to reduce any anxiety, and he did not feel the need of any other help. When seen after completing his examinations, he reported that – even with one exam which was more difficult – at no time did he feel more anxious than would be normal for someone sitting an important exam. SD did well with these exams and on the strength of his overall marks his tutor encouraged him to enrol for a PhD. At one-year follow-up, he was able to sit his finals without experiencing undue anxiety.

While this case may not be typical of the average voice patient because of the high levels of individual and family disturbance, the description of approaches to treatment clearly illustrates the value of careful analysis, detailed preparation, target setting and role-playing in complex cases where there are blocks to expressing feelings or conflicts over speaking out which are very common in psychogenic voice disorder.

SUMMARY

- Since we have seen in Chapters 1 and 4 that PVDs are commonly provoked by stress and anxiety, in order to treat the underlying cause of the voice problem, SLTs need to be confident in treating anxiety. This chapter provides the SLT with a range of cognitive behavioural options that they can draw on when treating anxiety.

- Before commencing treatment, the therapist should provide the patients with feedback on their formulation from assessment and give a rationale for treatment strategies, including explaining the model of anxiety. This chapter therefore begins by providing that explanation of anxiety and describes the psychological changes (thoughts, feelings and behaviours) and physical changes that people experience when anxious.
- In order to treat anxiety in psychogenic voice disorder patients using CBT, the therapist needs to know how to:

  o teach physical relaxation techniques and rapid stress control
  o encourage self-observation as well as acceptance of anxiety
  o set appropriate targets
  o help the patient develop skill in challenging thinking errors and with developing positive self-statements
  o use cueing devices or prompt cards to facilitate new learning
  o use role-playing as a way of practicing specific cognitive behavioural skills.

These strategies are described for the SLT and it is recommended that the voice therapist acquires a level of competency and familiarity of using these strategies through clinical supervision or formal training.

8 Treating Lowered Mood in Voice Patients

A BRIEF INTRODUCTION TO THE NATURE OF DEPRESSION

Anyone who has ever experienced voice loss, however fleeting, will know how frustrating aphonia or dysphonia can be. Trying to speak and producing no voice at all, or just a whisper, can easily fuel irritation and anger. Not knowing what is wrong or what to do to make it right, as well as trying to speak and being unsuccessful, also evoke feelings of helplessness. Helplessness about not being able to understand or change a situation is associated with lowering of mood, appetite and energy levels, as well as an increase in negative thoughts and feelings of apathy, all of which are symptoms commonly found in depression (see Seligman 1975; Abramson et al. 1978).

Loss of physical abilities and losing something usually taken for granted such as the ability to speak and be understood, can also lower mood and cause depression. Psychologically, the person has to accept new limitations as well as the fact that they are not as invulnerable as they might have thought. There may even be times when an experience of loss of this sort becomes a symbol to the person of vulnerability or personal mortality and if this occurs it will cause even greater distress and grief (see Yalom 1980).

Because of these psychological processes, we would expect that many voice-loss patients suffer from lowered mood or symptoms of mild-to-moderate depression. Furthermore, we are now beginning to understand how loss of voice emerges in the context of stressful life events. Stressful life events are also known to trigger lowered mood or depression. For these reasons (i.e. reacting to voice loss and/or reacting to an external stress causing dysphonia), the client's mood is likely to be low when they attend for voice therapy.

Psychological research is now making it clearer as to the way in which lowered mood influences how we think about ourselves and our world and how normally positive and optimistic people find their thinking becomes negative and pessimistic as a result of feeling down in spirits (see Teasdale 1988 and Segal et al. 2002 for a review). It seems that when something happens to cause negative thoughts and to lower mood, we then begin thinking negatively about other things as well. This then drags our mood even lower, potentially pulling us deeper and deeper into depression. To make things worse, in a depressed state of mind there is a common tendency to distort the truth about ourselves, for example, to minimise our successes and magnify our failures. This is why cognitive therapies have focused on helping the person catch and challenge these cognitive distortions and find more reasonable, fair, realistic and rational (hence more positive) ways of thinking. The assumption is that not giving in to or dwelling on negative thinking will boost their mood and then begin to alter their depression.

The Challenge for the Speech and Language Therapist:

The challenge for the voice therapist working with some patients with psychogenic voice disorder will be knowing:

1. how to recognise signs of lowered mood;
2. how to access the associated negative thoughts;
3. how to offer practical ways of fighting negativity in order to elevate mood.

At the same time, we must stress that we do not expect the SLT to shoulder the responsibility of treating a patient's depression. If patients show noticeable signs of depressed mood they should always be referred to a specialist for treatment.

However, because lowered mood or depression will be found associated with voice loss, we believe that a better understanding of depression and treatment strategies improves outcome for many voice patients.

NOTABLE COGNITIVE FEATURES OF LOWERED MOOD

When people become depressed they get caught up in very powerful, negative beliefs about their own worth and the value of their past achievements. They may also see their world as a place that, with few exceptions, is uninteresting or meaningless, unpleasing or even painful, and a place where effort goes unrewarded. To make matters worse they find it difficult to believe that the future will bring any change to how they see things in the present. Thus, the days ahead are seen as an unending repetition of failing to achieve their standards or ambitions, and a distressing round of unrewarding and meaningless activities. Because of this common pattern in depression, the therapist should note the negative views the person describes about their self, their world, others, and their future.

Second, the therapist will observe that the negative cognitions of depressed patients are usually all-inclusive or pervasive across many or most situations. This contrasts with anxiety disorders where negative cognitions tend to be related to specific situations. For example, people who suffer from social anxiety may experience negative thoughts about themselves only when they have to confront a social situation. By comparison depressed people tend to dwell on what they consider to be their inadequacies and *any* challenge – personal, social, educational, professional – may trigger a string of negative thoughts.

Third, a common preoccupation of depressed people revolves around the theme of loss. They feel they have either lost or will never gain something that would make their life worthwhile or rewarding.

Fourth, of the many cognitive distortions that are found in depression, one of the most common is **selective abstraction**. This is a tendency to select out from the whole only information that supports a negative viewpoint. For example, in thinking about the past, they tend to select out from their total life experiences only their moments of failure and errors of judgement. As can be easily imagined, overly focusing on these selected experiences will support and reinforce their view that they are failures.

Finally, it is also common for depressed individuals to spend long periods of time ruminating about their condition (for example, wondering 'Why me?' or 'What have I done to feel like this?') and to be constantly comparing their current emotional state to a more ideal or happier state of mind. They commonly try to 'think their way out of depression' by looking for causes or endlessly going over explanations and, understandably, are usually preoccupied with trying to control or change their very distressing emotional state.

QUESTIONNAIRES

The questionnaires that cognitive therapists find most useful in assessing symptoms of depression and depressive thoughts are the self-scoring version of the Dysfunctional Attitude Scale (DAS: Burns 1980); the Hospital Depression and Anxiety Scale (HADS: Zigmond & Snaith 1983); the Beck Depression Inventory (BDI: Beck & Steer 1987) and the Young Schema Questionnaire (Young & Brown 2003). The BDI is an excellent, easily administered and brief scoring device for measuring the presence of depression and changes during or following treatment. The DAS and Schema Questionnaires, in their different ways, enable the therapist to focus on specific schemas that may underlie the depressive mood.

DESCRIBING THE COGNITIVE MODEL OF LOWERED MOOD AND DEPRESSION

Before beginning treatment the patient must be given a clear description of the cognitive model of depression so that they can appreciate the rationale behind a number of therapeutic activities. This will also foster compliance and motivation with homework, etc. The therapist may find that hand-outs developed by Powell (2000) are helpful for this purpose.

TREATMENT STRATEGIES

The first 11 points in a list compiled by Williams (1984) of treatment components in cognitive behaviour therapies are of relevance in treating depression:

1 teaching self-monitoring of activities
2 teaching self-monitoring of mood
3 teaching self-monitoring of thoughts
4 (graded) task assignment – teaching how to set appropriate goals

5   teaching self-evaluation of behavioural achievement; mastery and pleasure techniques

6   teaching self-reinforcement for behavioural achievement

7   teaching thought-catching and how to identify themes and assumptions in thought content

8   teaching 'distancing' of thoughts by labelling as 'hypotheses'

9   teaching how to evaluate evidence for 'hypotheses' (reality testing)

10 teaching how to deal with implications of thought evaluation

11 teaching how to find alternative rational responses to negative thoughts

Further components of cognitive behaviour therapy listed by Williams such as 're-attribution training' and 'teaching how to increase formerly or potentially pleasant activities', also have a role in working with depressed patients. In the rest of this chapter we will describe the most common or core treatment strategies used in the treatment of depression.

TEACHING SELF-MONITORING OF ACTIVITIES, MOOD AND THOUGHTS

Teaching self-monitoring of activities, mood and thought is usually achieved by encouraging the daily completion of an appropriate record sheet. As a general rule the therapist should start with a simple record sheet (Table 8.1) and make the record-keeping more complex as therapy gets under way (Tables 8.2 and 8.3).

The record sheet shown in Table 8.4 illustrates the thoughts, thinking errors and healthy challenges recorded by a young dysphonic woman who suffers from lowered mood. She is in a relationship with a man who is very controlling and, at times, unthoughtful of her needs. At the time of being asked to keep a thought record she is thinking of taking the step of confronting her partner over his tendency not to consider her needs. This is followed by an alternative record sheet (Table 8.5), which collects information that will be valuable in the therapy session. This final record sheet helps capture the process of thinking and feeling. With practice patients should become more able to challenge their initial interpretation of a situation. Hopefully, this should lead to a positive emotional change.

TASK ASSIGNMENT AND GOAL SETTING

In asking the patient to keep daily record sheets the therapist is also taking the first step in task assignment and teaching how to set appropriate goals. The first task is to keep the record. The goal is to gain insight into patterns of negative thoughts, when these are triggered and how they affect mood states or motivation. With the ongoing assessment of dysfunctional cognitions and behaviour as therapy unfolds, new targets or goals will emerge.

The other components of CBT (points 5–11 listed above) and more recent therapeutic developments overlap somewhat and would usually be focused on through specific strategies. These can be illustrated under the following headings.

Table 8.1: Daily record sheet #1

Daily Record Sheet		
Date	Situation/Activity	Thoughts

Table 8.2: Daily record sheet # 2

Daily Record Sheet			
Date	Situation/Activity	Negative Thoughts	Positive Alternatives

Table 8.3: Daily record sheet # 3

Daily Record Sheet

Date	Situation/Activity	Negative Thoughts	Belief in Thoughts Rated 1–10	Positive Thoughts	Belief in Thoughts Rated 1–10

Table 8.4: Record sheet # 4

Record sheet		
First (Unhelpful) Thought	**Thinking Error**	**Second (Helpful) Thought**
1. If I say what I think, he won't accept it and he'll be critical and angry.	1. Jumping to conclusions.	1. I don't really know that he won't accept it or how he'll respond till I tell him how I feel.
2. But why bother speaking to him, I never do anything right, anyway.	2. Overgeneralisation.	2. That's nonsense. There are lots of things I get right and do well.
3. But it won't be any good doing it if I can't say everything I want to say.	3. All-or-nothing thinking.	3. It doesn't have to be perfect. It's important to make a start not to do it perfectly.
4. But it never comes out the way I want to say it so I'm bound to mess it up, say the wrong things, and make things worse.	4. Overgeneralisation. Jumping to conclusions.	4. I usually say things as I want to say them. I'm not necessarily going to mess up or make things worse.
5. But even if I speak to him, he always has the last word, so I can never win.	5. Jumping to conclusions. All-or-nothing thinking.	5. So what? That's not important. Anyway, maybe this time will be different. Expressing my feelings is what's important. Besides, all this has nothing to do with winning or losing. It's simply about asserting myself and letting him know how I feel.
6. But I know that if I speak my mind and tell him what I think and what I want, he'll leave me.	6. Jumping to conclusions.	6. I don't *know* this. Even if he doesn't like what I say it shouldn't be a reason for leaving. By speaking my mind he might actually start to respect me more.

ELICITING THOUGHTS IN THE THERAPEUTIC SESSION

The ability of any individuals to observe dysfunctional thoughts will depend on their ability to be 'mindful' and introspective. They need some degree of psychological sophistication and they may also be influenced by their acceptance of the cognitive approach as a way of understanding and solving their problems. However, people usually can be helped in this endeavour by these therapeutic strategies:

1   The therapist can explore and analyse a recent situation triggering negative cognitions and causing emotional distress. This can be done in the first interview when taking the history or in later sessions by asking patients to elaborate on their daily record sheet.

Table 8.5: Record sheet # 5

Daily Record Sheet

Situation/Activity	Emotion and Intensity 0–10	First Thoughts	Alternative Thoughts	Believability of Positive Thoughts 0–10	Emotion and Intensity 0–10

2   If patients appear emotional when recounting certain events, ask them whether they are aware of any particular thoughts causing the feeling.
3   Patients can be encouraged to recall the most recent event causing a change of mood. Ask them to visualise the scene and recall the specific thoughts they were having at the time.
4   The therapist will employ the Socratic questioning and downward arrow techniques described on pages 46–7.

WAYS OF EXPLAINING THINKING ERRORS

Throughout any session the therapist should help patients search for a new perspective, asking them for alternative interpretations of how they look at things, enquiring if there might be a way of re-attributing the cause or the outcome of events. For example, in the case of harsh self-criticism, the therapist should find an opportunity to ask if patients are applying a double standard in their thinking. Patients can be asked to consider how they would react if a good friend described similar failings? 'In the same circumstances would you be more sympathetic with a friend than you are being with yourself?' 'Is your problem that you're too hard on yourself or don't know how to be kind to yourself?'

Another helpful strategy can be using an analogy to highlight an error in thinking. For example, the therapist might compare a tendency to overgeneralise to someone doing badly in a preliminary test and not bothering to sit later exams. A similar analogy might be to comment that if one piece of fruit in a bowl is bad you don't throw the lot away.

The analogy of seeing a partially filled glass of water as either half-empty or half-full can be particularly useful with some patients. For example, Grace, an elderly patient with Reinke's Oedema, was referred to the first author because she was also chronically depressed. Being widowed, isolated and having a poor relationship with her grown up children, she had many things about which to feel depressed, but the assessment of her daily thoughts showed that she was most often preoccupied with sad thoughts about her grandson. Some years ago she had made contact with a daughter who had been placed in care when Grace was 18. Through the reunion she became particularly close to her daughter's teenage son who came to live with her in London and had promised always to stay living with Grace. However, after several years together, he moved into his own flat. Although he lives locally, telephones most days and regularly visits Grace, she continues to feel very hurt by his failure to keep his promise to always live with her. For Grace, the analogy that she was seeing her glass as half-empty rather than half-full was particularly helpful as an image of the way she was letting a loss and disappointment colour how much she still had and how lucky she was to continue having such a good relationship with her grandson. By recalling the image of the half-full glass, Grace was able to develop a means of fighting the sad feelings that arose when thoughts of her grandson came to mind.

Sporting analogies are often valuable. For example, a patient who was seen in ENT with serious loss of hearing following an ear infection and who had become depressed, commented to her psychologist that an additional factor fuelling her lowered mood was a difficulty she had forming relationships with men. Due to the fact that her father, her ex-husband and an ex-partner had all taken her for granted or made her feel used, she found she had become very intolerant of men. In describing this she spontaneously used a sporting analogy: 'If they make one mistake or do one thing wrong that's it. It's like "one strike and you're out."' She agreed that she needed a way of thinking that was less extreme if she wanted any future relationship to work. The therapist pointed out that she was looking for a more flexible, less all-or-nothing, way of thinking and suggested extending the sporting analogy to soccer where for minor misdemeanours the referee shows the player coloured warning cards before finally sending him off the pitch.

Some errors of thinking can be highlighted by showing how they are exaggerations of reality and if they are followed to their logical conclusion are quite absurd. This can often be done with a touch of humour. For example, patients holding the belief that they are unlovable because they are unattractive or ugly could be cajoled with statements such as 'So if you're as bad as you say, then people would be aghast to see you. They'd point and turn their heads in horror and rush from the rooms you enter. Showmen would have asked you to appear in their circus or sideshow. The government would have even passed laws to stop you terrifying children!' Even with very depressed patients this usually raises a smile of acknowledgement.

PROVIDING INFORMATION ABOUT DYSFUNCTIONAL THOUGHTS

While most patients quickly grasp the connection between negative thoughts and lowered mood, they usually need some guidance to fully appreciate the type of thinking error they are making. As illustrated earlier in the record sheet example in Table 8.4, it is possible for patients to identify the type of thinking errors they are making or the type of traps into which they are falling. This example shows commonly observed thinking errors such as **all-or-nothing thinking** where anything short of perfection is considered a failure or of no value; **overgeneralisation** where the person believes one error or failure shows that they are never successful in anything; and **jumping to conclusions** where they assume they know that others are thinking negatively about them or that they are going to respond negatively toward them in the future. (See Burns 1980, for a detailed description of these and other cognitive distortions.)

We find it helpful to use the following hand-out (adapted from a sensitivity check list in Juniper 1978) to provide both information about cognitions and lowered mood and a systematic way of analysing thoughts and feelings:

IDENTIFYING THE PSYCHOLOGICAL CAUSES OF FEELING DEPRESSED

In fighting depression it is important to learn to observe and identify your depressive thoughts and feelings; to understand why they have emerged; to assess whether you are making a particular type of thinking error; and, finally, to think of ways to challenge unhelpful beliefs and attitudes.

In defeating depression, it will be helpful to see thoughts and beliefs as theories that should be abandoned if they are found wanting or inadequate; to see them as only *one* way of looking at things. Get into the habit of observing and challenging or questioning your tendency to think in a certain way. Consider alternative conclusions. Remember, depression feeds off wrong conclusions. The following check list will help you analyse your thoughts and feelings in a systematic way. It can be a helpful reference or guide if you are keeping a daily record of situations and thoughts that provoke depressive feelings.

SENSITIVITY CHECK LIST

STEP 1: BEGIN BY ASKING YOURSELF TO IDENTIFY THE THOUGHT AND FEELING

1   What is the depressive feeling?
2   Is it accompanied by a depressive thought or image?
3   What was happening when I first thought this way?
4   Is this an area in which I am particularly sensitive?
5   Have I thought in this precise way before?
6   Are the circumstances the same as on that previous occasion?

STEP 2: ASK YOURSELF WHAT TYPE OF THOUGHT AND FEELING THIS IS

Having identified the thought that precedes the feeling, try to clarify it in one of the following categories, asking yourself whether it is associated with:

1   Low self-esteem.
2   Ideas of deprivation/self-pity (e.g. 'Nobody likes me', 'I am alone', 'unlovable', 'unwanted', etc.).
3   Self-criticism/self-blame (e.g. 'It's all my fault').
4   Overwhelming problems/duties (e.g. 'I can't cope', 'It's all too much', etc.).
5   Self-commands (e.g. 'I must do so and so', etc.).
6   Escapist and suicidal wishes (e.g. wanting to withdraw, run away, or thoughts of killing yourself).

STEP 3: ASK YOURSELF IF YOU ARE MAKING A PARTICULAR SORT OF THINKING ERROR

To answer this question analyse the thoughts in more detail.

1   Am I jumping to conclusions?
2   What is the evidence for my conclusions?
3   What is the reason or reasons for feeling like this?

4   How strong is the evidence?
5   Is there an alternative interpretation?
6   Am I being over-selective and ignoring another, broader view of things?
7   Am I overgeneralising? For example, am I saying that one mistake means I never perform well or that I am a complete fool?
8   Have I made any exaggeration of minimisation of my performance? In other words, am I making a wrong estimation of my performance?
9   Have I labelled the activity or situation inaccurately or made a wrong interpretation?
10 Are there other ways of interpreting the event or is it possible to draw a more positive conclusion? For example,

   Am I concentrating on my weaknesses and forgetting my strengths?
   Am I blaming myself for something that is not my fault?
   Am I taking something personally, which has little or nothing to do with me?
   Am I expecting myself to be perfect?
   Am I using a double standard – how would I view someone else in my situation?
   Am I paying attention only to the black side of things?
   Am I overestimating the chances of a disaster?
   Am I exaggerating the importance of events?
   Am I fretting about the way things ought to be instead of accepting and dealing
   with them as they come?
   Am I predicting the future instead of experimenting with it?

TEACHING HOW TO SET APPROPRIATE GOALS AND HOW TO EVALUATE OUTCOME

Because patients with lowered mood can find it very difficult to motivate themselves and also tend to undervalue their successes or interpret their efforts as failures, it is extremely important to help them set appropriate goals. At all stages a goal must be easily attainable. An example might be agreeing to phone a friend for a chat that does not focus on gloomy subjects. The therapist must also let the patient know that although under normal circumstances this might be an easy thing to initiate and carry through, the lowered mood will make it both hard to do and difficult to appreciate or value what is actually achieved.

Goal setting can also provide an opportunity to help the patient observe and challenge negative thoughts that feed passivity (e.g. 'What's the good of trying that? It won't make any difference') or thoughts which reduce positive feelings about the effort they have made (e.g. 'I found it hard to think of things to talk about. He didn't seem to want to talk for long. Who'd want to talk to me, anyway?'). If patients have not already done so, the therapist will need to help them reframe their thoughts and explore more positive conclusions. Here the therapy should be helping the patient learn how to view their efforts more realistically and rationally. They should also be learning the important cognitive behavioural rule that not rewarding or actually punishing yourself through negative thinking leads to lowered motivation and mood, while rewarding yourself through such things as self-praise and positive, rational thinking, improves motivation and mood.

TEACHING MINDFULNESS AND MINDFUL ACCEPTANCE

In recent years research by Teasdale (1988); Teasdale et al. (1995); Teasdale et al. (2000); and Segal et al. (2002) has shown that individuals who experience recurrent episodes of low mood are often drawn more deeply into a state of depression because of factors such as (a) ignoring or being unaware of changes in both mood and thinking (being on automatic pilot or not being fully in the present moment); (b) focusing a lot of mental effort on trying to get rid of their negative emotions and inadvertently intensifying these feelings; (c) endlessly ruminating about current and desired states of mind; and (d) relying too much on their ability to think their way out of depression. Following on from their research, these same psychologists have explored the value of training individuals in acceptance and mindful awareness to counter these tendencies. The intention of the training has been to help individuals become more aware of times of a potential relapse into depression, to teach them how to live more fully in the present moment, how to accept or hold uncomfortable feelings without resistance, how to disengage from ruminative patterns of thought, and how to shift to another, non-thinking, state of mind. A one-year follow-up of a large random control trial with patients who had suffered from recurrent episodes of depression indicated that this approach approximately halved the rate of relapse (Teasdale et al. 2000; Segal et al. 2002).

While we do not expect speech and language therapists to necessarily have the skills or time to take patients through a full training programme of acceptance and mindful awareness, we feel it is important that they stress to patients the value of becoming aware of the negative effects of rumination and attempts at emotional regulation. Put another way, one role of the therapist should be to help patients see the value of being mindful of their current mental/emotional state and accepting of (rather than struggling with) their involuntary emotions. For example, having in early treatment explained the rationale for being mindful, for not ruminating and not struggling with negative feelings, it takes only a few minutes to ask in later sessions how well they are doing at noticing and stepping out of ruminations about their condition or mood, and how well they are getting on at not resisting or pushing away negative feelings.

BEHAVIOURAL EXPERIMENTS

Behavioural experiments are experiments that are developed collaboratively between the therapist and patient. The aim for patients is to predict the outcome they would expect if they carried out a certain action. Patients then agree to carry out the action and to evaluate the results. For example, a dysphonic patient who fears expressing opinions might say, 'I haven't the courage to speak my mind to my husband because he'll dismiss my views out of hand and then I'll feel low and rejected and more depressed than I do at present.' Having explored and challenged these assumptions cognitively and, perhaps, role-played or rehearsed the situation in the session, the therapist and patient agree on a behavioural experiment to test her predictions. As a result, the patient finds that she does have the courage to express what she feels, that her husband listens to what she has to say, that he does not reject her and that she feels more self-confident rather than depressed.

Behavioural experiments and behavioural strategies can provide a powerful means of cognitive change. In fact, a study by Bennett-Levy (2003) suggests that setting behavioural experiments may have more impact on outcome than focusing treatment on cognitive strategies like keeping automatic thought records. In this study participants, being trained to use both automatic thought records and behavioural experiments, reported that with their therapist's support and encouragement the behavioural experiments had more impact on their thinking and were more powerful and compelling in changing beliefs and behaviour than the analysis of automatic thought records.

SETTING TARGETS THAT SHOULD MAKE LIFE MORE REWARDING

Finding ways of helping patients make their lives more rewarding is a major feature in the cognitive behavioural treatment of depression. In fact, some authors go so far as to emphasise that making life more rewarding (or increasing positive reinforcement) is the single most important factor in decreasing feelings of depression (Azrin and Besalel 1981). The following list outlines some ways in which the therapist can encourage patients to increase the rewards in their lives through setting targets. The list can be given as a hand-out but the therapist will need to guide and elaborate as well as take patients step-by-step through the 14 targets because depressed patients need a lot of encouragement to work consistently at these goals.

FIGHTING FEELINGS OF DEPRESSION BY MAKING LIFE MORE REWARDING

The following list (originally from Azrin and Besalel, 1981) describes 14 behavioural strategies designed to fight depression and make life more rewarding. The list suggests initiating a number of new or neglected activities which should be positively reinforcing and should boost positive feelings.

1 Maintain contact with others. (Depressed people tend to withdraw from social contacts but often forget their depression when socialising, particularly if distracted from self-preoccupation.)

2   Keep active. There are many physical and mental benefits from increasing activities when feeling depressed: it distracts us from selfpreoccupation, increases alertness, reduces feelings of lethargy, improves mood and self-confidence and provides a sense of physical and mental wellbeing. Do not let more than two days go past without involving yourself in at least a 15–20 minute period of exercise that makes you breathless. Even a brisk walk can be helpful. Keep a chart of activities to help motivation.

3   Consider ways of finding the right balance in work and leisure.

4   Regularly remind yourself of achievements (e.g. jogging, telephoning friends).

5   Make a roll call before sleeping of the day's accomplishments.

6   Follow a strict rule of never adding 'ifs' and 'buts' when reviewing achievements and accomplishments.

7   Write down all the qualities you like about yourself. Ask family and friends to tell you the qualities they like in you.

8   Make a list of people you like and why you like them.

9   Regularly praise yourself by practising statements from your list of qualities you value in yourself. Add this to your evening roll call.

10 Make a list of things that gave you *happiness, pleasure* and *interest* in the past.

11 Set daily and weekly targets to engage in rewarding activities. (Use the list of things that have given you happiness as a guide.)

12 Try and have a daily conversation with someone where you deal *only* with pleasant topics of mutual interest.

13 Make a list of bad things in your life which contribute to your depression and compile a list of things that have not been affected. Add this to your reviews of pluses in your life.

14 Check the list of objectives and targets weekly to assess progress.

Guidelines for the Speech and Language Therapist

If therapists feel the need for further guidance in creating an activity chart, activity planning and rating, as well as suggestions for listing pleasant activities and goal setting, they will find it helpful to consult the self-help hand-outs developed by Powell (2000).

SUMMARY

Lowered mood or depression may be triggered by stressful life events that underpin PVD, furthermore voice disturbance itself may evoke feelings of helplessness which can contribute to lowered mood. Therefore, in order to effectively manage the voice patient, this chapter aims to equip the SLT to have an understanding of depression together with CBT treatment strategies.

Check list of assessment and treatment techniques used in treating lowered mood and depression

- Look for the presence of negative views about self, world, others and future.
- Note that pervasive, all inclusive negative thoughts are common.
- Look for a common theme of loss in what is being described.
- Look for the tendency to select out from the whole only that which suggests a negative point of view (**selective abstraction**) as it is one of the most common cognitive distortions in depression.
- Use appropriate questionnaires to assess depression.
- Provide the patient with a description of the cognitive model of depression.
- Teach self-monitoring of activities, mood and thoughts.
- Focus on assigning tasks and setting appropriate cognitive behavioural goals.
- Elicit thoughts in the therapeutic session.
- Explain thinking errors within the therapeutic session.
- Provide written and verbal information about dysfunctional thoughts including

  - definitions of cognitive distortions
  - identifying the psychological causes of feeling depressed
  - sensitivity check list.

- Teach how to set appropriate goals and how to evaluate outcome.
- Encourage mindfulness and mindful acceptance.
- Make use of behavioural experiments to challenge beliefs.
- Set targets to make life more rewarding.
- Employ the hand-out *Fighting Feelings of Depression by Making Life More Rewarding* as a step-by-step guide.

9 Psychological Disorders: Deciding When Not to Treat

Because voice loss may appear in association with a particular psychological condition, knowledge of different disorders can help when assessing treatment possibilities and when considering referral to a psychologist or psychiatric specialist for an opinion. The most important conditions you will need to consider will commonly fall into one of five broad categories: **anxiety disorders, somatoform disorders, personality disorders, affective disorders,** and **schizophrenic disorders.** In this chapter we will give a brief description of each disorder, showing how they have been understood by contemporary psychology and mentioning the sort of treatments they might require. We will not attempt to cover everything in detail – just what we feel might be most important to know about.

Although we will describe the disorders separately, it should be stressed that there is often an overlap between different categories and within the subgroups. From a CBT point of view, the important thing about considering these classifications is that it enables the assessor to think sympathetically and comprehensively about the type of problems the patient is experiencing. This leads naturally to considering how best to apply appropriate treatment techniques or to considering whether certain signs indicate that a disorder may require input from another specialist.

ANXIETY DISORDERS

Depending on the type of symptom, anxiety states can be classified as **generalised anxiety, phobic anxiety, panic disorder, post-traumatic stress disorder,** or **obsessive-compulsive disorder.** The person suffering from an anxiety state will report experiencing a variety of symptoms. The following check list should be helpful in recognising an anxiety state:

- o 'butterflies' in the stomach;
- o physical restlessness or agitation;
- o physical tension or difficulty relaxing;
- o impatience, distractibility, irritability, feeling 'wound up' or 'on edge';
- o intrusive negative thoughts or worries;
- o difficulty getting off to sleep;
- o bad dreams or nightmares;
- o waking in fear at night;
- o feelings of apprehension or dread;

o dry mouth;
o clammy hands or excessive bodily sweating;
o feeling light-headed, faint or dizzy;
o rapid pulse;
o pounding heart;
o diarrhoea;
o a lump in the throat or difficulty swallowing;
o frequent micturition;
o fears or phobias;
o attacks of panic;
o obsessional thoughts and/or compulsive behaviour.

The presence of anxiety will be the most common of the psychological conditions seen in the voice clinic and the SLT will find it invaluable to understand the various forms it takes and to be familiar with treatment strategies.

GENERALISED ANXIETY DISORDER

The person suffering from generalised anxiety persistently experiences anxiety and feelings of panic in a wide variety of situations. It has been described as 'free floating anxiety' because it often occurs unpredictably or without the sufferer being able to explain the cause of the anxiety. The psychoanalytic view is that this is because the underlying cause of the anxiety has been repressed. Biologically-oriented psychologists suggest that the temperament or autonomic nervous system of sufferers is more sensitive to change, stimulation and stress, causing them to overreact to the challenges of life. Behavioural psychologists assume that the anxiety is being stimulated by classically and operantly conditioned associations. Cognitive psychologists look for hidden schemas and anxious predictions that provoke feelings of fear. The SLT will usually find that offering anxiety management techniques will benefit individuals with generalised anxiety.

PHOBIC ANXIETY DISORDER

In phobic anxiety, feelings of fear are attached to a particular object or situation. The fear is intense, irrational and will usually lead to avoidance behaviour. The irrational nature of phobic reactions can be seen most clearly when the anxiety attaches itself to common, everyday objects and situations: certain foods, birds and insects, going into open spaces, using the telephone, socialising, being alone in the house, etc.

Freud believed that phobias are formed as a defense against an unconscious, psychological conflict (see Davison & Neale 1982, for more details). Contemporary psychology does not entirely reject this interpretation but takes the view that phobias are mainly learned anxiety reactions. Put simply, the person has, for one reason or another, become anxious while in the presence of a particular object or animal or situation and the anxiety reaction has been reinforced and maintained through the principles of classical and operant conditioning. For example, a woman feels trapped in a supermarket because of the crowding and long queues, she panics and runs out. On her next visit to the supermarket the same conditions evoke negative (classically conditioned) associations, including feelings of panic, which cause a repeat of the avoidance behaviour in an effort to reduce the anxiety. The decline of the anxiety will reinforce or reward the avoidance response and establish (through operant conditioning) a pattern of avoidance behaviour. As suggested by this example, phobias are associated with the person feeling physically or psychologically vulnerable and with instinctive survival reactions – such as the fight-or-flight or startle response – being triggered. While this suggests that phobias are not directly caused by unconscious conflicts in the way suggested by Freud, some phobic reactions, such as panic attacks when staying away from home and agoraphobia, do appear to mask or reflect the deeper, unconscious or only partially-conscious fears, for example, an unresolved separation anxiety (Butcher 1983) or fear of death (Butcher 1984). Cognitive therapists have also shown that *catastrophic thoughts* (for example, thoughts of fainting, dying, making a fool of yourself) can be triggered by *the physical sensations of anxiety*, and this, commonly, intensifies a fear reaction (Clark 1986,1996; Salkovskis and Hackmann 1997). When phobic reactions lead to intense panic, as in the condition of agoraphobia, it is now common practice to consider that the condition is a symptom of **Panic Disorder**.

Systematic desensitisation (Wolpe 1958) is an effective treatment for many phobic conditions, although CBT has been used successfully in treating more complex phobic reactions like agoraphobia (Salkovskis and Hackmann 1997; Hackmann 1998). Since the treatment of phobias will usually fall well outside the role of the Speech and Language Therapist, we recommend referring to a clinical psychologist in most cases. However, a knowledge of stress management and self-instructional training, along with graded exposure or changing safety behaviours will be invaluable in treating those voice disorders associated with social phobic anxiety.

PANIC DISORDER

Patients suffering from anxiety disorders often report having attacks of intense, uncontrollable panic that may be triggered by certain situations but often occurs in an apparently spontaneous way. The prevalence of panic symptoms and the fact that the panic is often viewed by sufferers as the primary and most distressing symptom, has led many clinicians to use the term **panic disorder** to highlight that this is a unique or separate condition within the anxiety disorders. However, the term panic disorder is controversial (see, for example, Gath and Goeting 1990). Many clinicians argue that it is not a separate disorder in itself but a symptom that can develop within general anxiety and phobic anxiety states. It is assumed that anyone suffering from high levels of anxiety would be more prone to panic attacks due to the fact that anxiety levels are nearer the point at which states of panic can be triggered. Thus, a particular life stress may cause someone with mild anxiety to become moderately anxious, while someone with moderate or high levels of anxiety might experience a panic attack or a series of panic attacks. If not treated, these may become habitual. Some phobic conditions such as agoraphobia are considered a panic disorder because unexpected and unpredictable panic seems to cause and maintain the condition but, as we described above, the panic can usually be traced to conditioned associations (e.g. feeling trapped) and to catastrophic thoughts (e.g. 'I'm going to die') evoked by the physical sensations of anxiety.

From the perspective of your assessment, the important thing to take into account will be whether the patient describes panic symptoms. These symptoms will indicate the presence of high levels of anxiety, more severe problems and a more challenging treatment proposition. Whenever panic disorder is indicated, it will be sensible to seek the collaboration of one of the mental health specialists.

POST-TRAUMATIC STRESS DISORDER (PTSD)

The distinguishing feature of this anxiety disorder is that it follows a major and traumatic life event or life events involving actual or threatened death or serious injury or a threat to the psychological integrity of oneself or others (e.g. rape). It can result from a reasonably brief, single event such as a serious accident, a natural or man-made disaster, or a protracted experience of fear or series of life-threatening events such as those experienced by soldiers in combat. In PTSD the person has been exposed to serious personal threat or, as in the case of combat veterans, has lived through periods of time expecting death or injury to themselves while witnessing the death and mutilation of others. Symptoms commonly found in PTSD include general anxiety, restlessness, distractibility, phobias, panic, disturbed sleep, nightmares, flashbacks (intrusive images relating to the trauma or the traumatic events), avoidance of stimuli associated with the trauma, lowered sex drive and personality changes such as becoming moody, disinterested, cynical, pessimistic, and socially withdrawn or actively exhibiting antisocial behaviour.

Psychological explanations of PTSD (e.g. Smucker 1997) relate the condition to the shocking nature of events that are so outside normal experience that the person has difficulty making sense of what has happened and coming to terms with it, psychologically. Phenomena like flashbacks are seen as attempts by the mind to process and to find a way to come to terms with the traumatic experience. It is likely that temperament and personality factors make some individuals more prone to developing PTSD after a traumatic event.

Patients suffering from PTSD will be rarely encountered in a voice clinic. However, the condition with voice loss can be triggered by trauma to the throat or an experience of nearly choking to death. For example, we have described in detail a case of a man who became dysphonic, had difficulties swallowing food, and showed many classic symptoms of PTSD when he nearly choked on a piece of sharp metal hidden in the food he was eating (Butcher et al. 1993). Cases of this sort require input from a clinician experienced in the treatment of PTSD.

The work of Baker (2003) with patients who have a psychogenic voice disorder that has been triggered by events associated with an earlier trauma is relevant here. This is described more fully in Chapter 1 (pp. 19–21). These presentations of PVD are rare.

In Baker's experience and interpretation the patient, unable to make sense of the horror of the event, becomes dissociated from the traumatic event and is therefore unable to recall it. We would advocate that where the SLT suspects that the voice disorder may be linked to an earlier traumatic event of that order, then the SLT should treat the voice disorder within a framework of clinical supervision from a clinical psychologist. That supervision may lead to referral to the psychologist.

OBSESSIVE-COMPULSIVE DISORDER

Individuals with this anxiety condition may suffer from either obsessional thoughts or compulsive behaviour but more usually they suffer from a combination of these cognitive and behavioural symptoms. A person suffering from obsessional thoughts experiences recurring unwelcome, unacceptable or bizarre and distressing thoughts and images that intrude into consciousness. The thoughts are often about breaking social taboos such as becoming violent or sexually disinhibited or simply saying something that would bring embarrassment or social disapproval and can, thus, be related to concerns about impulse control.

The thoughts are usually overvalued in the sense that the person feels *responsible* for the thought or the action suggested by the thought. For example, a mother may have a thought or image of being careless and harming her child. Most mothers would assume this arose out of concerns for their child or would dismiss it as just a thought, but an obsessional person would tend to interpret the thought as a clear indication that they are careless and likely to harm their child. Trying not to dwell on such an unacceptable thought and trying to repress it has the paradoxical effect of making the thought return more frequently. The woman may then become completely preoccupied or obsessed with the thought of being a dangerous or bad mother. Often in these cases the obsessional person feels that having the thought is the same as actually committing the action. Thus, having an image about harming your child becomes as awful and distressing as having physically carried out the act.

Someone showing symptoms of compulsive behaviour feels compelled to carry out repetitive actions. These actions are usually *attempts to rectify an unacceptable or undesirable error* (e.g. repeated checking of gas, light switches, door locks, or something the person has written) or *attempts to reduce fears about contamination* (repeated washing to avoid germs or dirt, feeling infected or unclean).

Thus, individuals with an obsessive-compulsive disorder (OCD) are often motivated by fears of loss and change and criticism and the wish to achieve order, control and perfection. Their compulsive behaviour may also reflect irrational, phobic concerns about threats to physical safety. In addition to these symptoms, some individuals also find their mental and physical processes slowed down, a condition known as **obsessional slowness**. In these cases it can take the person an inordinate length of time to complete even simple tasks.

Obsessive-compulsive disorder is equally common among men and women and one of the rarer psychiatric conditions (0.3 and 0.6% of psychiatric outpatients according to Rachman and Hodgson 1980). It generally emerges in late adolescence and early adulthood in individuals of above average intelligence whose personalities tend to be perfectionistic, cautious, conscientious, rigid and parsimonious.

The different psychiatric, psychoanalytic and psychological explanations of OCD have in common the view that there are constitutional personality factors (such as neuroticism and introversion or a predisposition to rigidity and perfectionism) that usually underlie the condition and which are aggravated by anxiety-provoking life experiences associated with order, success, perfection, personal control and safety. (For a review, see Rachman and Hodgson 1980; Salkovskis 1989; and Shafran 1999).

Although OCD is a rare condition, patients with obsessive-compulsive tendencies or personality may present for treatment in a voice clinic. Because of their personality or obsessive-compulsive problems they can be either very conscientious in carrying out treatment instructions or noncompliant due to the distraction of intrusive thoughts and/or compulsive rituals. Psychologists have developed a variety of cognitive-behavioural techniques to treat obsessive-compulsive problems (e.g. Salkovskis 1989; Holland 1997). Therefore, the more chronic or difficult to treat obsessive-compulsive with a voice disorder should always be referred on to a mental health specialist for further help.

SOMATOFORM DISORDERS

Somatoform disorders are conditions in which the body (or soma) is the focus of symptoms. In these cases the individual complains of a physical symptom, or combination of symptoms for which no physical cause can be found. The symptoms also appear to meet unconscious needs to elicit sympathy and caring from others or to avoid particular activities. The somatoform disorders have been categorised as **conversion disorder, somatisation disorder, psychogenic pain disorder** and **hypochondriasis**.

Two other conditions with a psychological element that have a somatic focus are **chronic fatigue syndrome** and **irritable bowel syndrome**. Many clinicians believe that chronic fatigue is a symptom of depression and that it should be included in the range of depressive disorders, while a majority would classify irritable bowel syndrome among the anxiety disorders. Whatever the merits of classifying these conditions in these ways, for our present purpose we feel that it makes more sense to discuss these fairly common conditions in this section because the patient's and therapist's focus will be on the somatic features of the condition.

CONVERSION DISORDER

With a conversion disorder the individual experiences a physical dysfunction for which there is no evidence of organic pathology. Symptoms include loss of visual, verbal or auditory function, loss of ability to feel touch or experience pain, and paralysis or partial paralysis of limbs. A conversion disorder usually emerges in the context of life stress and speech and language therapists will most commonly encounter conversion disorder in the form of psychogenic, functional, or non-organic voice loss.

Freud first proposed the psychoanalytic view of conversion disorder in 1896 (see Freud 1962). He suggested that repressed energy associated with the sexual or aggressive instincts is *repressed* and *converted* into a physical symptom which, in an important way, directly symbolised the essence of the inner, *unconscious*, conflict. While Freud made a number of modifications to his original theory (see Barskey 1989), he always retained this essential formulation of conversion disorder and stressed how the condition is maintained by **repression** and **primary and secondary gains**. The repression effectively removes the inner conflict and the anxiety it causes, hence the patient presents with *la belle indifference*, little motivation to fully engage in therapy and may appear resistant and controlling. In more recent times social, cultural, developmental, behavioural and cognitive behavioural models have been employed in attempts to explain conversion disorders from a non-analytic view point (see, for example, Davison and Neale 1982; Butcher 1995).

We have outlined our views on the conversion model in relation to understanding psychogenic voice disorder in Chapter 1. In brief, we have argued that the majority of patients with psychogenic voice loss – the group we have called Type 2 – appear to be suffering from symptoms of musculoskeletal tension and anxiety caused by life stress and interpersonal conflicts that frequently involve difficulty in expressing feelings. While distress is converted into a physical loss of voice and while inhibited anger may play an important role, these feelings are consciously accessible to the patient. These patients are suppressing their emotions; there is no repression operating and therefore no presence of *la belle indifference*. Because of these features, these Type 2 conversion patients do not otherwise fit comfortably into the Freudian interpretation of conversion disorder. Whatever the diagnostic challenges confronting the therapist, the important thing for the SLT to keep in mind is that there is good evidence that voice therapy with the Type 2, more common, form of psychogenic voice disorder can be enhanced by incorporating psychological treatment strategies (e.g. Butcher et al. 1993). Also, as we explained in Chapter 1, where a classical Freudian conversion (or as we describe it, a Type 1 conversion) is suspected, the SLT should refer to a psychologist or psychiatrist for support in confirming the diagnosis.

SOMATISATION DISORDER (BRIQUET'S SYNDROME)

Individuals with this syndrome describe *multiple* physical symptoms which greatly restrict their life but for which no organic cause can be found. They experience a *variety* or *combination* of physical symptoms including fatigue, nausea, blurred vision, weakness, aches in joints or back pain, burning in the mouth, rectum or vagina, headaches, chest pain and dizziness. In a study of patients diagnosed with this condition, Perley and Guze (1962) found that 44% suffered from aphonia and 28% reported experiencing a lump in the throat. Thus, patients with this disorder may present in a voice clinic. The more pathological or chronic forms of this disorder have much in common with the extremely challenging Type 1 conversion disorder, in that their emotional conflict appears to be unconscious. These types of patient have proven difficult to treat with psychotherapy. However, we should note here that the majority of patients describing a lump in their throat (*globus pharyngeus*) will not be suffering from Briquet's Syndrome but have most similarity with Type 2 conversion patients who suffer from psychogenic voice loss (for example, showing features of emotional over-control and difficulty expressing feelings) and there is little doubt that some globus patients do benefit from a combination of voice therapy and a psychological focus in therapy (Mathieson 2001, p.221). The important thing, therefore, is to keep in mind that although more frequently presenting as a single symptom of stress, or accompanying a voice disorder that will be amenable to treatment in the voice clinic, globus may sometimes present as part of multiple somatic symptoms (Briquet's Syndrome) and will be more resistant to therapy.

CHRONIC FATIGUE SYNDROME

From time-to-time, the SLT might also find that, along with the voice problem, their patient complains of somatic symptoms associated with **chronic fatigue**. The experience of chronic fatigue is one of extreme tiredness and loss of energy, often with aches and pains, rather as if the person never recovers from a major viral infection. There is still debate over whether the fatigue has its origin in a viral infection but, whether this is a factor or not, a frequent finding is that people with chronic fatigue symptoms have become caught in a cycle of overactivity, exhaustion and taking extended periods of rest to recuperate. Since the inactivity leads to a decline in fitness this becomes another complicating factor. Many sufferers are people who find it difficult to put limits on the physical and social demands in their life. Thus, the moment they feel a little more energetic they overdo things and exhaust themselves or set themselves back. If they rest too much they become more unfit and more easily exhausted when next trying to be more active.

Since taking on too much and overdoing things is also common in psychogenic voice patients, there may be times when they present in the clinic with symptoms of chronic fatigue. In these cases, the therapist will find it valuable to suggest target setting in order to reduce commitments and to also help the patient develop a philosophy of monitoring and pacing activities, rest and energy expenditure. This is similar to the behavioural approaches, like prescribing voice rest or restricting noisy social events, which are commonly used in voice therapy and the therapist should feel at ease in extending the treatment focus to cover other stresses that may be affecting outcome. As many therapists also introduce graded exercise as a way of increasing stamina and fitness, the SLT may wish to seek guidance from another professional such as a physiotherapist who is experienced in this work.

IRRITABLE BOWEL SYNDROME

Patients may also be seen who complain of somatic symptoms such as stomach pain and diarrhoea that are commonly diagnosed as **irritable bowel syndrome**. Since this particular condition is typically aggravated by anxiety and stress, patients may gain indirect benefit from the stress management techniques that are used in treating their voice. However, while there is good support from research to show that CBT is effective in treating chronic fatigue, the evidence is mixed with irritable bowel syndrome as to the benefits of relaxation training and cognitive behaviour therapy. (See Raine et al. 2002, for a review of treatment outcome with chronic fatigue and irritable bowel syndrome.)

PSYCHOGENIC PAIN DISORDER

Patients complain of severe, protracted pain for which no physical cause can be found. Often this is in one part of the body. For example, a sufferer may approach his or her dentist because of a continued burning sensation in the mouth or may present in the ENT department complaining of a similar pain in the throat. Like other somatoform disorders, the condition may occur or worsen in the context of life stresses, may provide the person with a reason for avoiding a particular activity, and may be evoking the attention and sympathy of others. *Globus pharyngeus* may also fall into this category of illness if the sensation is experienced as particularly painful. Many sufferers from psychogenic pain disorder get a degree of relief from training in relaxation and distraction techniques but the more challenging cases may need to be referred to a clinical psychologist or psychiatrist for treatment.

HYPOCHONDRIASIS

In this condition, the individual is preoccupied with their health and symptoms that, in their mind, suggest they have a life-threatening illness. For example, a headache or dizziness is interpreted as a brain tumor, palpitations become a heart attack, and abdominal discomfort suggests bowel cancer. Individuals with hypochondriasis tend to have anxious personalities. From a cognitive perspective it is now well established that an individual who is anxious or depressed will tend to interpret events (including bodily changes/symptoms) in a negative rather than in a positive or unconcerned way.

Sufferers are not easily reassured by a medical consultation and will return again and again to their general practitioner or Accident and Emergency departments of their general hospital with the same symptoms. If symptoms decline, the person usually becomes over-preoccupied with new symptoms of what is perceived to be another life-threatening disease. Although the SLT will often find their patients express fears that their voice loss is an indication of a serious physical illness, particularly cancer, this is a perfectly understandable anxiety and not hypochondriasis in the true sense of the word. The difference can be judged by whether the patient's anxiety reduces with information giving and reassurance about the true nature of the symptoms. The truly hypochondriacal patient will continue to hold on to the morbid belief and fail to be reassured. Treating hypochondriasis is difficult and requires an experienced specialist (Warwick and Salkovskis 1989; Sisti 1997). Referring on or collaboration with a specialist is always advisable.

PERSONALITY DISORDER

Although taking several extremes, the general features of personality disorder are impaired, inflexible and maladaptive social and occupational functioning. These individuals have commonly had traumatic, often brutal, and insecure early histories that have made it difficult for them to develop appropriate attachments to others and a personal sense of identity. The following lists some common features found in personality disorder:

1. Poor reality testing – lost in unreal or escapist fantasies; confused identity or having exaggerated views of their own importance, showing poor judgment of what is normal or acceptable.
2. Lack of conscience – the presence of antisocial behaviour and a tendency to live on the wrong side of the law or on the fringes of society.
3. Difficulties with relationships – poor empathy or little feeling for others; may be charming on the surface but this is in the cause of self-interest and exploitation of others; at one extreme can be paranoid, at the other dependent, and frequently showing problems in recognising appropriate interpersonal boundaries.
4. Unpredictable, violent moods, impulsive or reckless behaviour.
5. A need to seek stimulation, excitement or attention.
6. May display traits of perfectionism and passivity that mask anger and aggression.
7. Poor self-image may manifest as low self-confidence and over dependent behaviour.

Because of their poor reality testing, difficulty with relationships and impulsive or thoughtless behaviour, patients with personality disorder find it difficult to comply with or learn from treatment. This being said, and while accepting that this is an extremely difficult population to treat, there have been promising results using CBT with individual cases (Beck et al. 1990; Padesky 1994) and where the resources are available to offer intensive, long-term treatment with either cognitive behavioural (Linehan 1993; Arntz 1994) or psychoanalytically oriented therapy (Bateman & Fonagy, 1999). However, even highly experienced mental health workers find that patients with a personality disorder are some of their most demanding and challenging clients. (For a description of the difficulties of treating a voice patient with personality disorder see Butcher and Elias 1983.) Thus, when your assessment indicates the presence of symptoms or behavioural patterns typical of personality disorder, it is advisable to make an early referral to a psychiatrist or clinical psychologist.

AFFECTIVE DISORDERS

It is quite common for people to experience one or more changes of mood in the course of a day. Usually, these mood swings are quite minor. For some people, however, mood swings are more extreme and their mood can plummet into depths of **clinical depression** or lift to heights of intense elation or **hypermania**. These mood states may be

bipolar (encompassing both episodes of depression and mania) or **unipolar** (taking the one extreme of mania or, more commonly, depression).

MANIA (OR HYPERMANIA)

It is extremely rare for individuals to suffer from mania without experiencing a period or periods of depression. Thus, mania is usually one extreme in a bipolar (manic-depressive) disorder. An individual in a hypermanic state can be easily recognised by:

1. having an elevated, elated, expansive mood;
2. being excessively talkative, often with an abnormally fast rate of speech;
3. shifting rapidly from one topic to another (a phenomenon often referred to as *flight of ideas*).
4. displaying increased energy and physical activity levels;
5. sleeping less than the usual amount;
6. becoming easily distracted or diverted from one train of thought or activity to another;
7. showing inflated self-confidence and self-esteem, exaggerated, unrealistic views of self-importance, abilities or talent;
8. behaving in disinhibited and reckless ways such as going on spending and gambling sprees and being sexually promiscuous.

A full-blown episode of mania will require psychiatric input and is usually treated with hospitalisation and tranquillisers. Psychological approaches are largely ineffective at these times. Manic episodes are usually stabilised over time by prescribing *lithium carbonate*. When a person's mood state is normal or more stable, he or she can be trained to watch out for early warning signs of mania and to take steps that might inhibit the manic state. For example, noticing they are taking on more and more work, setting over-ambitious deadlines, sleeping less or burning the candle at both ends socially, he or she will note these warning signs and try to target behaviours that reverse the trend toward a manic episode (see Lam et al. 1999). Although there may be an opportunity for psychological therapy as described, for example, by Lam et al. 1999, and while in these cases it may be valuable to make suggestions about monitoring over-activity, etc., rarely, if ever, would offering psychological treatment to individuals coping with a manic disorder be a role for the SLT.

DEPRESSION

The distinguishing features of depression can be listed as follows:

1. lowered mood state experienced as sadness or depression, accompanied by feelings of hopelessness and meaninglessness;
2. thinking dominated by negative, self-critical, suicidal thoughts and feelings of guilt, blame, unworthiness;

3. sluggish thoughts, indecisiveness and disturbances of concentration;
4. decline in energy and feelings of fatigue;
5. difficulty summoning up normal motivation or interest;
6. decline or loss of interest in activities which normally give pleasure;
7. changes in activity levels: being moderately or inordinately slow at tasks or demonstrating signs of physical agitation;
8. changes in appetite and weight: usually a decline in desire for food and loss of weight but appetite and weight may be in the opposite direction;
9. changes in normal sleep pattern: insomnia, early morning waking, or sleeping excessively.

In some cases, patients experience a combination of depressive and anxiety symptoms. In severe clinical depression thinking can become bizarre and unrealistic to the point of appearing psychotic, for example, having the delusion of being guilty for all the sins of the world. Fortunately, the more common forms of depression are less severe.

Research in the 1970s and 80s suggested that cognitive therapy for patients with mild-to-moderate depression is as effective as pharmacotherapy in reducing the depression and also appears to make the person less likely to relapse in the months following treatment (Rush et al. 1977; Kovac et al. 1981). While, as Gelder (1990) points out, more recent research has questioned this last point and indicated that, in terms of preventing relapse, cognitive therapy is not superior to maintenance doses of antidepressants, 'there are individual patients in whom relapse seems to be closely related to cognitive or interpersonal problems and in these cases psychological treatment can be tried when other measures have failed' (p. 1088). More recently, mindfulness-based cognitive therapy (MBCT) has been shown to significantly reduce relapse in major depressive disorder (Teasdale et al. 2000).

Mild-to-moderate depression is the most likely to be encountered in the voice clinic. While it would not be advisable for the SLT to attempt to treat a patient who is seriously depressed, milder forms of depression associated with voice loss may be tackled as an adjunct to voice therapy provided the therapist has grasped the treatment principles outlined in Chapter 8 of this book and has received supervision from an experienced or accredited cognitive behaviour therapist.

SCHIZOPHRENIA

Schizophrenia is more common than OCD but not as common as anxiety and depressive disorders. Apart from being reasonably rare the disorder can be so disruptive of normal patterns of thought and behaviour that the person is unlikely to present in the outpatients of a speech and language therapy department. However, the condition does create disturbances of speech – particularly poverty of speech and blocking. Although these relate to disturbances of thought processing, they are of some interest to the speech therapist/pathologist. In the rare event of someone with schizophrenia attending in a voice clinic it will be necessary to distinguish these speech problems from more common forms of voice loss or speech impediment and to recognise the need to make a referral to a department of psychiatry for assessment. In some ways the diagnostic task is made easy by the oddity or strangeness of the symptoms, which are typically what most people think of as madness.

The main disturbance in schizophrenia is in thought or thinking. This can manifest itself in a number of ways that are associated with a variety of emotional and behavioural changes.

1. Thinking processes appear (a) easily distracted, (b) incoherent or disordered, (c) illogical, (d) ungrammatically bizarre and with (e) far-fetched or loose associations.
2. Speech may include (a) made up words (**neologisms**), (b) nonsense phrases (**clang associations**), (c) the persistent repetition of ideas (**perseveration**), (d) disruption or stopping or tailing off before finishing a sentence (**thought blocking**), and (e) noticeable reduction in the usual amount of normal speech or the content conveying little or no information (**poverty of speech**).
3. A characteristic feature of schizophrenia is the presence of **delusions** and **lack of insight** into the condition. The delusions are commonly of a **paranoid** nature and include (a) distorting or misreading the significance of everyday events (for example, believing that someone scratching their nose indicates something important or sinister), (b) believing that their thinking is being interfered with, that their thoughts are being broadcast to others or an external force is either taking their thoughts away or inserting thoughts that are not their own, (c) that their emotions are being controlled, and (d) that their impulses, actions or somatic sensations are the result of an external agent or force.
4. Perceptual distortions often take on the quality of an **auditory hallucination**. Usually, this is an external voice that repeats their thoughts, comments on a situation or criticises other people or their own action. In marked contrast to the popular stereotype of madness, visual hallucinations are rare.
5. Affective symptoms can be particularly striking, with mood being (a) unresponsive to stimulation or invariably flat and apathetic or (b) showing **inappropriate affect** such as laughing during a sad occasion or becoming enraged or giggling for no good reason.
6. Disturbances in **motor activity** commonly include bizarre facial expressions, odd, often repeated movements and gestures of limbs, or with hands and fingers, either showing an increase in motor activity or decrease to the point of long periods of frozen immobility or **catatonia**.

Psychiatric treatment for schizophrenia employs neuroleptic or antipsychotic drugs. Psychological treatments such as family behaviour therapy (Falloon 1985) have been shown to prevent relapse and cognitive behaviour therapy can help reduce symptoms (Meichenbaum & Cameron 1973; Chadwick & Birchwood 1994; Garety & Freeman 1999).

As can be seen from the above description, schizophrenia is a complex and highly challenging condition. Although eminently treatable with psychological approaches (see for example, Chadwick & Birchwood 1994), schizophrenia requires the sort of time and special experience that falls outside the role of a speech and language therapist working in a voice clinic.

WHEN TO TREAT AND WHEN TO RE-REFER: A SUMMARY

ANXIETY DISORDERS

The various anxiety disorders can all be treated with CBT (e.g. Beck & Emery 1985). Anxiety will present as a common feature in the voice clinic and guidelines for treating general and mild anxiety conditions are described in Chapter 6. The treatment of phobic anxiety, panic disorder (with or without agoraphobia), PTSD and OCD involves using techniques that are more specialised and time-consuming. Therefore, as a general rule, these conditions will require the expertise of an experienced cognitive behaviour therapist and should be referred on.

SOMATOFORM DISORDERS

Some somatoform disorders respond well when treated with voice therapy in combination with CBT, particularly the conversion disorder that makes up approximately 95% of psychogenic voice disorders that we have labelled Type 2 conversion (see Chapter 1). Patients with psychogenic pain disorder can benefit from learning stress management skills and training in distraction techniques, while hypochondriacal patients can be helped through using cognitive challenging and restructuring to change their interpretations of bodily symptoms (see the case examples on pp. 181–200 of this volume). However, these treatments can be difficult and time-consuming and, as with other complex conditions, we advise referring psychogenic pain and hypochondriacal patients on to a specialist.

The SLT will often find there is a role in offering help to somatisation patients, particularly those who suffer from aphonia and from *globus pharyngeus*. Treatment of somatisation conditions in the form of chronic fatigue and irritable bowel may also be offered in the clinic but only as an adjunct to treating the voice and as part of teaching life and stress management skills. In all these cases, it is perfectly appropriate for the SLT to provide a therapeutic lead, but we expect that given how challenging these conditions can be, there will often be times when the therapist will need a second opinion or will need to refer to a mental health specialist.

PERSONALITY DISORDER

The treatment of personality disorder is very much the province of an experienced therapist. Thus, we always recommend re-referral whenever your assessment suggests the individual is suffering from features of personality disorder.

AFFECTIVE DISORDERS

Mania

If a patient is well when seeing a speech and language therapist but has a history of hypermania, the SLT may want to offer suggestions or guidance on, for example, being mindful of increasing activity levels or hypomanic behaviour (an early stage of hypermania) and taking appropriate steps to slow things down if this occurs. However, the SLT should immediately consult a specialist if the patient is showing signs of becoming hypermanic.

Depression

We do not recommend that the speech and language therapist attempts to treat anyone who is seriously depressed. Given, however, that lowered mood often accompanies psychogenic voice disorder, Chapter 8 of this volume provides an introduction to techniques that can be helpful in treating mild-to-moderate depression and can be used as an adjunct to restoring voice and in helping the patient return to normal.

SCHIZOPHRENIA

While psychological approaches have been of proven benefit in cases of schizophrenia, this is a challenging, time-consuming population, and one that requires input from an experienced specialist. Therefore, we recommend that the SLT always refer these patients on for a psychiatric assessment.

> **In all cases when first initiating CBT forms of treatment, we recommend that the SLT is supervised by an experienced or accredited cognitive behaviour therapist.**

SUMMARY

Knowledge of psychological conditions can help in assessing treatment possibilities and the need to refer to a specialist. The different types of psychological conditions have been broadly classified as follows: **anxiety disorders**; **somatoform disorders**; **personality disorders**; **affective disorders** and **schizophrenic disorders**.

ANXIETY DISORDERS

These can be recognised by the presence of common symptoms (see pp. 157–8) that may become manifest in the following ways: **generalised anxiety** (where anxiety emerges in a wide variety of situations); **phobic anxiety** (the intense irrational fear of a specific object or situation); **panic disorder** (predominant and/or spontaneous, uncontrollable panic attacks); **post-traumatic stress disorder** (an anxiety state following a serious threat of death, injury or loss of physical and personal integrity to self or others); and **obsessive-compulsive disorder** (the experience of intrusive, unwanted thoughts and compulsive behaviours).

SOMATOFORM DISORDERS

The somatoform disorders come in four 'types': **conversion disorder** (where psychological distress is converted into a physical symptom); **somatisation disorder** (which has a lot in common with conversion disorder but is a condition where the patient complains of a variety of physical symptoms, aches and pains); **psychogenic pain disorder** (an experience of medically undiagnosed, severe and protracted pain in one part of the body); and **hypochondriasis** (the interpretation of bodily sensations and minor symptoms as signs of serious illness where the patient is not reassured by consulting a specialist).

PERSONALITY DISORDERS

Common general features are impaired or maladaptive social and occupational functioning. This is related to poor reality testing and poor self-image. There are notable difficulties with relationships. These difficulties develop out of having formed maladaptive attachments in early life and from, for example, making perfectionistic demands of others while finding it impossible to set personal boundaries, being impulsive, having unpredictable mood swings, craving for stimulation or attention, and expressing overly dependent or independent behaviour.

AFFECTIVE DISORDERS

These disorders include the polar extremes of **hypermania and depression**. Manic states involve elevated mood, inflated self-confidence, high levels of energy and activity and difficulties maintaining trains of thought. Depression usually shows itself in lowered mood, decreased appetite and activity levels and changes in the content of thought that becomes dominated by negative, self-critical views, hopelessness and suicidal feelings.

SCHIZOPHRENIA

Schizophrenia is most easily recognised by various types of delusions (particularly and more commonly of a paranoid nature), descriptions of auditory hallucinations, disturbed affect and disturbances of behavioural or motor activity. Someone suffering from this condition is unlikely to present in a department of speech and language therapy even though the sufferer may experience speech problems due to disturbances of thought processing.

WHEN TO TREAT AND WHEN TO REFER

Since all conditions may require the help of an experienced cognitive behaviour therapist or other mental health specialist, a basic understanding of psychological disorders and an idea of when it is best to re-refer will be of value in the voice clinic. Anxiety disorders, somatisation disorders, personality disorders, affective disorders and schizophrenic disorders have all benefited from cognitive-behaviour therapy. However, some conditions, for example, personality disorder and schizophrenia, are more difficult to treat or need more intensive and long-term therapy from a specialist in the field. For this reason, it is not really appropriate for the SLT to consider taking a treatment lead in these cases.

As a general rule, we believe that with appropriate training and supervision SLTs should consider treating the anxiety and lowered mood states that accompany psychogenic voice disorders as well as using CBT with relevant conditions within the somatoform disorders or, for example, when presented with chronic fatigue. However, when confronted with other, more challenging psychological conditions, they should refer these patients to a mental health specialist.

Initially, psychological treatment should be under the supervision of an experienced or accredited cognitive behaviour therapist, with the SLT working more independently with experience.

10 Case Studies

To conclude this book we offer a number of case studies of psychogenic voice disorders that illustrate the three types of conversion described in Chapter 1 and a contrasting muscle misuse dysphonia. It is hoped that these case studies will provide example of the diagnostic features that distinguish each type of conversion as well as describing management techniques that include both symptomatic voice therapy and cognitive behavioural therapy. In some of these cases the authors have worked independently with the patient and in others they have collaborated. The case studies show some of the challenges for speech and language therapists when working with psychogenic voice disorders but also some of the rewards.

DIANA: TYPE 1 CLASSICAL HYSTERICAL CONVERSION DYSPHONIA

PRESENTATION

Diana was a 46-year-old school teacher who arrived in the Combined Voice Clinic as a second opinion from a neighbouring area. She had become suddenly dysphonic 10 months earlier and had been in a persistent falsetto voice since that time. Many sessions of symptomatic voice therapy had failed to restore her to modal voice. The referring SLT reported being able to achieve some normal voice in intoned exercises and humming but this was not sustained in conversation. The SLT could not identify any psychological factors contributing to this voice disorder.

In the voice clinic the SLT was able to facilitate short glimpses of modal voice from a laugh and a gliding vowel and Diana was able to visualise her healthy larynx. Apart from expressing some frustration with her voice she did not exhibit any anxiety or lowered mood. She struck the voice clinic team as being rather emotionally 'bottled up' and despite some gentle questioning she denied having any life stresses or worries. She did not show any self-reflection and seemed to externalise the voice disorder, demanding, 'what's my problem?' and 'when will it return?' The SLT offered Diana two sessions of voice therapy to see what might be achieved.

PSYCHOLOGICAL ASSESSMENT

In the first lengthy session the SLT worked symptomatically but also attempted to obtain a more detailed psychological profile and case history. Diana was married with two teenage children; she could not identify any difficulties, stresses or changes at home. She had worked as a primary school teacher for many years and until quite recently had been happy at work. She did say that prior to her voice loss she had had a disagreement with the headmaster and had argued with him, although she did not elaborate and she gave the impression that she thought this was rather irrelevant. On the way to school 10 months earlier she clearly remembered the voice change. Since that time she had been unable to work and following a more recent referral to her Occupational Health Department she was considering early retirement. She seemed to be ambivalent about her job and she displayed no anxiety at having been off work for almost a year. Thus the SLT felt that she was probably benefiting from some secondary gain. The SLT found the psychological interviewing with Diana challenging as she remained dismissive of a connection with life events/stresses and the SLT was left with no avenues to follow.

Although the connection between life stresses and the voice was explained, Diana was primarily given a physical explanation of the voice disorder and the SLT said that she would help Diana's throat muscles to release from the faulty habitual pattern that they had established. This was the least challenging approach for Diana, and the SLT was left feeling that she was doing all the work. Diana's mood was upbeat, she smiled and laughed in the clinic but offered little input and the SLT felt she was rather detached from ownership of the voice problem and was expecting the therapist to fix it.

Diana's larynx was held firmly high and tight, although interestingly she felt no muscle ache or discomfort. The SLT palpated the laryngeal muscles firmly and the subsequent session Diana did report being aware of some temporary aching after the session. Diana was compliant with voice exercises. The therapist worked through a series of body, breath, and voice exercises with Diana lying, sitting and standing. Normal modal voice was achieved and this could be extended into phrases so long as it was intoned, but as soon as it moved to speech the tight, falsetto dysphonic voice returned.

Diana then cancelled two subsequent appointments and, although she gave reasonable excuses, this left the SLT feeling irritated and taken advantage of. The SLT had prioritised the sessions for Diana and had scheduled them at some personal sacrifice in her busy diary before taking a summer holiday. When Diana did attend for her second session the outcome was much as before. Modal voice could be achieved in exercises but not in speech tasks, and Diana remained detached from any personal responsibility for her voice leaving the therapist feeling controlled and irritated. The SLT took Diana calmly but firmly through a series of voice exercises and at one stage light-heartedly said that she was having to be a bit of a bully to help things to change. Diana retorted bluntly and loudly, 'you won't be able to bully *me*!' A suggestion made to Diana in the first session that she may like to consider investing in a session or two with an osteopath – specialist in voice disorders – was turned down in the second session on the grounds of expense especially since she was now on half pay from work. Although this was an entirely valid reason, it surprised the SLT who had reasoned that a short-term financial outlay might achieve a longer-term financial investment if it resulted in helping to regain her voice and a return to work. It struck the SLT that there was little evidence here of a motivation to return to work.

Having made no progress the SLT took supervision from a clinical psychologist. This enabled the SLT to clearly see the strong features of a Type 1 conversion in this case. It was hypothesised that the conversion into a debilitating voice disorder, which rendered Diana unable to work, was as a consequence of the repressed anger, or aggressive 'impulse', that she felt towards her boss. Effectively repressing this instinct allowed her to be free from any anxiety associated with this inner conflict. The subsequent denial of any stress, or of any self-insight or ownership of her voice problem had made her impossible to treat. This detachment, her *belle indifference* and resistance to any exercises that led to speech or suggestion of osteopathy, left the SLT feeling irritated and powerless. The SLT seemed to be working much harder for a resolution than the patient! This patient–therapist dynamic therefore reinforced Diana's original position: this was a physical problem that she expected the therapist to fix and she was more a bystander than fully engaged in the process. Given the difficulties with patients of this type, the psychologist felt that further voice therapy would be unproductive.

A difficult lesson for the SLT was the psychologist's suggestion that any number of SLT sessions would meet with similar resistance and his recommendation that she should discharge the patient. This suggestion was based on the fact that the features of the Type 1 hysterical conversion that the SLT had identified would make it difficult to work with this patient at either a psychological level or symptomatically. Being able to discuss the case and understand the psychological processes of a hysterical conversion was crucial in enabling the SLT to make the management closure decision for the case.

The SLT met with Diana to explain that as neither the previous voice therapy nor her recent therapy had been effective, that there was no advantage in continuing with this route. She reviewed the history of events with Diana and offered her hypothesis that the voice loss might have its origins in the argument she had had with the headmaster and therefore there was a psychological cause to her persisting difficulties. The SLT explained the link between loss of voice and repressed emotion. Diana rebuffed this angrily and made it clear that she found this interpretation unacceptable. After some discussion there was cordial agreement that whereas the SLT might maintain her view that a psychological cause was most likely, Diana did not share it. Diana agreed that in the therapist's discharge letter to the referring ENT Consultant, the therapist could state her opinion regarding the likely origin of the voice disorder but she could not be specific about a link with the headmaster – thus a compromise was reached. Finally, Diana displayed her usual cheerfulness and lack of anxiety and said that she had decided to follow up some other avenues of help, both homeopathy and a neurologist's opinion. The SLT and the patient left on good terms despite no change in Diana's symptoms.

CASE SUMMARY

This case illustrates key features of a Type 1 classical hysterical conversion as explained overleaf.

Predisposing factors

Little detailed personal history was obtained that might throw light on Diana's way of coping with unacceptable or threatening emotions especially dealing with expression of anger. However, there were suggestions in Diana's strong and dominant personality that made denial and repression a preferred coping mechanism. She showed no ownership for her voice problem and would not contemplate self-reflection. She was quite adamant that she could not be bullied, suggesting a strong or controlling personality.

Precipitating factors

The disagreement and argument at work with the headmaster preceded the voice loss. This suggests a conflict for Diana in her expression of anger with a key person in her life – the resulting dysphonia gave her a way out of having to express her anger or outrage. The conversion into a loss of voice may have symbolic significance as it occurred at the site of verbal expression.

Perpetuating factors

The repression operating in this Type 1 meant that Diana had effectively removed both the conflict from consciousness and all associated anxiety. Diana displayed no awareness of the conflict that had led to the conversion, nor any anxiety about the conflict or indeed any life stress. Neither did she exhibit any anxiety about her voice loss or her inability to work. She presented with typical *la belle indifference*, laughing and cheerful and with only mild frustration. The primary gain (removal of the conflict from consciousness) and the secondary gain (not having to work and the possibility of a retirement package) were sufficient to maintain the voice disorder. Diana's motivation for change was therefore low. This was demonstrated in many ways, specifically her cancelled appointments, refusal to consider osteopathy, and ultimately an inability to progress the voice exercises into speech. This behaviour all felt like resistance to the SLT who became irritated and powerless.

JOAN: TYPE 1 CLASSICAL HYSTERICAL PSYCHOGENIC VOICE DISORDER

PRESENTATION

Joan was a 53-year-old woman married 33 years, with three grown up children who had left home. She presented with a four-year history of dysphonia and intermittent aphonia. During voice assessment she was aphonic but was able to produce a cough. There were secondary difficulties associated with coping poorly with her voice loss. Neurological investigations, MRI scans, laryngeal EMGs and respiratory consultations all showed negative results and a three-month course of voice therapy failed to make lasting change.

PSYCHOLOGICAL ASSESSMENT

Joan presented as a small, timid woman with flattened affect and looking older than her 53 years. She was accompanied by her husband who sat quietly in the background and conveyed an impression of uninvolved weariness or boredom, of having been through all this before to no good effect.

Joan's scores on the HADS showed the presence of moderate depression and moderate anxiety. However, during the interview she denied currently experiencing unusual levels of stress. In terms of excluding a Type 2 diagnosis she also denied experiencing any conflicts over speaking out – saying she rarely holds back from speaking her mind – or carrying the burden of family responsibility – saying she can keep a distance from family problems and can talk to others about her concerns and dissatisfactions. At the same time, she did admit that her children come to her with worries and that she takes on their responsibilities, even to the point of sorting out their financial problems. When questioned about taking this responsibility as a possible burden, she denied finding it stressful. She gave the impression that she either enjoyed this role or thought it was what she should do as a good mother.

Throughout the assessment it became clear that Joan typically used repression or denial as a coping mechanism. This was most obvious when her voice problem began. She recalled that it followed a throat, eye and ear infection that began in May four years earlier. On exploring more about her life around that time she disclosed casually that a few weeks earlier in April she had seen her GP about a lump on her tongue. As a result of the consultation the GP arranged an urgent referral to her local hospital and two weeks later the lump was removed. She reported not feeling alarmed and could only recall that 'It happened very fast.' A series of open questions failed to illicit a clear picture of her thoughts and feelings about the lump and on directly being asked whether she thought she might have had cancer, she replied that she had 'not once thought of it being cancerous'.

A second example of her tendency to use repression or denial to cope with stress was also illustrated by Joan's reaction a year earlier to being teased about her voice by a work colleague. She described how she put up with it for ten days and how she felt it was 'something that really didn't bother me' until suddenly breaking down into uncontrollable tears and needing to take two days off work.

Similarly, although she admitted that her voice problem had been getting her down and that it affected her social life and other activities like answering the telephone, in general she denied being anxious and stressed – an emphasis that was contradicted by her high scores for anxiety and mild depression as shown on the HADS. The contradiction was partly resolved through questioning when it was found that Joan associated her high anxiety scores on the HADS (for example, worrying thoughts, restlessness, panic) with a fear of entering public places or being outdoors and said that she had been mugged twice in the past, and if it were to happen again she was now afraid she would be unable to call for help.

While this then becomes an interesting illustration of how anxiety can develop secondary to voice loss rather than being a cause of voice loss, there remains the apparent contradiction or paradox that the patient generally denies having had or currently experiencing stress in her life but is conscious of how some things are causing her anxiety. This contradiction can be resolved by suggesting that the defence of repression is only partial, generally working well to screen out anxiety and fear but failing to be effective in some situations or with some fears. Whatever the explanation, however, the important thing for the therapist to note is that this sort of presentation, with all its assessment difficulties and contradictions, is more typical in a classic Freudian (Type 1) conversion disorder and it suggests that repression is playing a major role in the voice disorder, restricting the patient's insight and making it difficult for the therapist to employ CBT or other psychological treatments.

CASE SUMMARY

This case of a middle-aged woman with aphonia illustrates the various symptoms associated with Type 1 psychogenic voice disorder. Although Joan's response to the HADS showed evidence of moderate anxiety and depression, she reported being unaware of experiencing any emotional stress. This suggested a tendency to repress emotional conflicts. In terms of excluding a Type 2 diagnosis she denied any difficulties in expressing her feelings. While admitting that her grown children do bring their problems to her and she takes on issues like sorting out financial problems that they should deal with themselves, she dismissed the suggestion that she was carrying family responsibilities. Again this indicated that Joan probably uses denial or repression as a mechanism of defence for coping with anxiety.

Joan's tendency to use repression is probably best illustrated by her response to having had to have an urgent operation to remove a lump on her tongue and, on another occasion, when being teased at work. In both instances she failed to recognise a level of emotional turmoil that for most other people would cause considerable distress. The presence of repression and lack of insight into her feelings are features that would make it difficult for Joan to use CBT as a means of overcoming her psychogenic voice disorder.

Schemas/personal beliefs/rules of living

Not known but some indication that she probably holds the belief that a good mother sorts out her children's problems.

Predisposing factors

Personality type that uses repression/denial as a coping strategy.

Precipitating factors

Developing a lump on her tongue which necessitated an urgent operation, followed shortly after by a throat infection.

Perpetuating factors

The continued use of repression and denial. Lack of insight. Possible secondary gains.

SARAH: TYPE 2 (COGNITIVE BEHAVIOURAL CONVERSION) DYSPHONIA

PRESENTATION

Sarah, a 37-year-old telephonist in a call centre, was referred to speech therapy with a 'normal larynx' and a six-month history of 'a warbling voice'. Her immaculate dress and smiling appearance gave no hint to the doctors of any emotional troubles. This outward appearance belied her inner sadness and vulnerability, which became apparent almost immediately during her voice case history and assessment.

Initially the SLT interview concentrated on the history of the recent increasing dysphonia. Sarah was a telephonist in a call centre and over the past three months had become aware of voice change and subsequent increasing difficulty in managing her job, so that she had been moved from telephone duties to paperwork. This inability to perform her job caused her great anxiety. The voice history then revealed that Sarah would typically lose her voice for a few days, about three times a year, when she had a cold. This had been a pattern for several years and although she reported this voice loss almost always accompanying a cold, she did say that occasionally her voice would go when she was upset – and in the absence of any URTI. Within the first tearful session her voice showed some variation. Habitually she was now using a falsetto quality voice with unstable pitch and at times rhythmical pitch breaks that resembled a tremor. However, after crying her voice was almost normal. There were no suggestions of vocal abuse, although she clearly was dependant on heavy voice use throughout the day.

In this first session Sarah was invited to speak a little about herself and to identify stresses in her life. She described typical tension sites in her neck, even when sleeping, poor sleeping patterns and panic attacks. She had been taking Prozac for six months. Sarah explained that she worried inwardly and spent a lot of the session crying silently. She readily began to discuss a little about her main areas of stress and unhappiness, mainly her work, which she hated; an unsatisfying relationship with a married man; and unresolved issues with her mother's death 10 years earlier and her estrangement from her father two years later. Sarah lived alone and although she said she did have friends she did not have confidantes and preferred to keep her problems and feelings to herself.

The therapist felt a great vulnerability and sadness from this lady. Outwardly she was working hard to put on a brave face – through her groomed and smiling appearance, and her deflection of the problem – because there are 'other people worse off than me'. However, her silent tearfulness and her readiness to confide in the therapist demonstrated the fact that she was suppressing a great deal of emotion and psychological stress. The assessment session was concluded by giving gentle feedback to Sarah; the SLT particularly reflected on the link that body tension has with the voice and, briefly, how emotions also contribute to that. The way forward suggested by the SLT was an offer of two to three sessions of therapy that would partly provide some practical help with Sarah's voice, some relaxation training and the suggestion that they may explore some of the emotions further. Sarah seemed grateful for the offer of help. From this initial session the SLT had in mind that this patient may require some formal counselling and possibly referral to a clinical psychologist.

In the second session the SLT reflected on the assessment with Sarah and how it had left Sarah feeling. She said that following that session she had been very exhausted but had subsequently begun to discuss some of her feelings with a friend. She also said that she had been troubled by bad dreams about her family and her mother, with a theme of Sarah feeling left out and alone. The therapist, sensing there was more to be told, explained that sometimes in order to look at the present it could be useful to explore some of the past. With no further prompting Sarah then told her story.

Sarah was an illegitimate child; she knew this from an early age and was referred to in the wider family as her mother's 'bastard daughter'. She thought her mother blamed her for taking away her youth. Her grandparents brought up Sarah while her mother worked. Soon her mother met and married a man that Sarah called her father. They had two boys, four years and six years younger than Sarah. The boys had some learning difficulties and she said they were given a lot of attention, whereas Sarah was given little attention and always felt isolated and unloved. She seemed to have learnt to look after herself early in childhood and she described herself as something of a Cinderella-figure in the family. She gave some vivid illustrations of this. For example, from the age of 11 years she was left at home to look after the animals while her parents and brothers went away for the annual summer holiday, but she longed for her mother to take her with them. She cried, childlike, while recounting this and other early experiences in the family.

Her mother had died in a road traffic accident ten years previously. Sarah had argued with her mother the night before. With her mother's death she felt she had lost her family. She said she was angry that her father was unable to manage any arrangements so she was left to identify the body, make the funeral arrangements and attend the inquest alone and unsupported. She then described an unhappy period at home. Her father became a changed man and fell to pieces, and Sarah was left to care for him and the brothers to a large degree. There had always been significant conflict in the family with rows and disagreements and the brothers had fought Sarah since their early teens. After her mother's death the violence escalated and Sarah no longer retaliated so that she was badly beaten. Eventually she left home and returned occasionally to do some chores. She felt that her father and brothers only wanted to have contact with her when there was something that they needed her to do for them. When her father began dating she found his girlfriend's place in her mother's home too difficult and she fell out with her father. She hoped her father would contact her but he never did, and this reinforced her view that she meant nothing to him.

Sarah spoke only a little about her boyfriend. She said, however, that she did not burden him with her problems. Since he was married, their meetings in her flat were arranged at his convenience and when he went home she was left feeling lonely and worthless.

Throughout this tearful hour-long session Sarah's voice was mostly normal. Following such a demanding session, it was important that the SLT give Sarah some feedback and to help her see the value and the way forward from so much disclosure. Sarah had some fair self-insight of the connections between the events and experiences in her life and her feelings of low self-esteem and lowered mood and she was congratulated on this insight and understanding. From the illustrations of her past, the therapist also reflected on her tendency not to voice her true feelings; for example, she said she had really wanted her mother to know how much she wanted to be asked to go on holiday, but instead she pretended she was happy to look after the animals. She was angry with her father after her mother's death because she was having to do all the coping at a time when she wanted to be looked after, but she did not express these feelings or her anger to her father. The therapist reflected on her ability to put on a brave face to the world, rather than disclose her real feelings to anyone. Against that backdrop of suppression of feelings, the therapist congratulated Sarah on being able to talk so fully about herself, and Sarah felt that had been a useful thing to do. The therapist suggested that they plan a couple of sessions to look at some of the immediate stresses with her voice at work, to teach some relaxation and stress management and to look specifically at adjustments to her voice and the work. The therapist explained the emotional link that the voice has with inner conflicts and with self-expression and she suggested that after a couple of sessions they should decide together whether the voice therapy sessions should be continued or whether Sarah might benefit from support from a clinical psychologist.

Voice therapy sessions focused on symptomatic therapy techniques, including some body relaxation, body release and vocal tract deconstriction as well as some specific advice for her work in the call centre and giving some attention to her emotional state. It was agreed after the two sessions that referral to a clinical psychologist, working in CBT, would be advantageous. The SLT arranged to continue with a few further sessions of voice therapy and then to review Sarah periodically. The therapy included some laryngeal palpation and work to reduce her habit of vocal strain. It was evident that she had a high level of muscle tension manifested in her neck and larynx, and any initiation of voice brought immediate and excessive tensioning in her extrinsic laryngeal muscles. The SLT continued to advise on modifications at work to support her voice including liaison with her occupational health doctor and employer.

Sarah subsequently reported to the clinical psychologist that she had been depressed on and off for a number of years and that this had developed gradually. Sarah reported that since taking Prozac she had generally felt more positive and less depressed, but her mood continued to fluctuate and some days she felt low and weepy. The clinical psychologist concluded that these difficulties had emerged in the context of generally negative self-esteem and increasing feelings of emotional isolation. The psychologist confirmed that Sarah was able to make links, with a fair degree of insight, between current problems and childhood experiences and relationships. Additionally, the psychologist identified that stress at work appeared to have been an exacerbating factor rather than an underlying precipitant to Sarah's distress. Finally, Sarah explained to the psychologist that she likened her current position to being 'alone on a raft' and that this represented both a position of safety and a position of emotional isolation.

The psychologist saw the link here with her adult relationships that had both been with married men, i.e. the fact that they are unable to make a commitment to her, or her to them, does not threaten her position of safety.

Sarah made good, steady progress. With the clinical psychologist she was able to explore and reach some resolution of conflicts arising from childhood experiences and gradually to feel less negative about herself and to develop self-esteem. Latterly in this process she began to express feelings of anger towards her mother, linked to her mother's behaviour towards her in her childhood. After a number of sessions, spanning in total a 12-month period, Sarah had made sufficient progress to feel happy for discharge from the clinical psychologist. Alongside this, Sarah changed her job and this alleviated the occupational stress on her voice. Sarah's voice was normal at this stage, but she had seen that fluctuations in her voice were influenced by occupational voice use, stress and emotional status. Sarah was discharged by the SLT at around the same time.

CASE SUMMARY

This is an example of a patient who has a predisposition to psychological problems as a result, primarily, of negative life experiences that had led to lowered self-esteem and feelings of poor self-worth. Since childhood she had been perceived as 'a coper' and was unaccustomed to speaking her mind or being assertive. In examining the inner emotional conflict it is possible to hypothesise that her poor self-esteem and her inability to express feelings made it impossible for her to express her anger to her mother for her emotionally deprived childhood. Her ongoing feelings of being value-less led to her unhappiness and depression. In keeping with her behaviour of keeping her feelings to herself, she gave an outwardly positive and attractive picture and did not share her conflicts and anxieties with anyone. She had therefore developed a strong coping mechanism of suppression, but her emotional stress continued and she suffered depression and many anxiety symptoms i.e. sleeplessness, panic attacks and muscle tension which focused especially in her neck, shoulders and larynx.

Recent work-based stresses added to her underlying stress. Her voice was vulnerable on two fronts: first, because she relied heavily on it for her vocally demanding job and second, because the anxiety, inhibition and physical tension around not voicing feelings was focused on the larynx. When her voice began to fail her and she became unable to do her job this provided some short-term secondary gain, in that she was given different duties, but this did not compensate for the distress it caused her nor did it change her unhappiness at work. Sarah's ongoing distress at an emotional level and her concern about her voice disorder led to good motivation to change and she was compliant and engaged in the therapeutic process.

Therefore, this patient can be confidently diagnosed as a Type 2 cognitive behavioural conversion dysphonia. Her dysphonia may have been precipitated by occupational stress and vocal misuse but the main driver (the predisposing and also the perpetuating factors) were the emotional conflicts related to self expression, assertiveness and self-esteem.

Predisposing factors

Early life experiences led to feelings of being unloved, valueless and therefore low self-esteem. She learnt early on to look after everyone else and not herself and not to express her needs or feelings. The unresolved issues with her mother (which were to a large extent repeated and reinforced by her stepfather and stepbrothers) and her feelings of poor self-worth led to a tendency to depression and a powerlessness to effect change. These factors predisposed Sarah to psychological distress.

Precipitating factors

Although upper respiratory tract infections coupled with her vocally demanding job were to some extent precipitating factors in her periodic voice loss and her current dysphonia, this did not explain satisfactorily her debilitating voice disorder. She did recognise that occasionally she would lose her voice in the absence of any cold and that her voice would deteriorate with stress. The precipitating factor in her dysphonia was likely to be the stress and unhappiness at work and her lack of assertiveness prevented her from expressing her unhappiness and finding a means of resolving these problems to her satisfaction.

Perpetuating factors

Sarah had not resolved her long-standing feelings of great unhappiness and loneliness, her anger towards her mother and stepfamily, or her feelings of loss of her mother. This meant that she continued to employ suppression as a coping mechanism and, as her inner conflicts were not resolved, she continued experiencing conversion symptoms. Furthermore, the unhappiness in the work-place and the high vocal demands of the job made it difficult to adopt good voice techniques, especially as she was suffering from so much excessive musculoskeletal tension.

JAMES: TYPE 2 (COGNITIVE BEHAVIOURAL CONVERSION) APHONIC TEENAGER

PRESENTATION

James was a 14-year-old lad who presented for a speech and language therapy voice assessment with aphonia, which had persisted following an upper respiratory tract infection some 10 weeks earlier. Although James attended for this first appointment with his mother, the therapist initially chose to see James alone, then his mother alone and finally the two together.

Despite whispering, James was a communicative young lad. He attributed his voice loss to a cold and inflamed tonsils. He reported some involuntary voice on the odd occasion, for example, when laughing and once when he swore because he had hurt himself. In the clinic he had a normal cough. These signs suggested that the voice was not strongly inhibited and when asked to perform voiceless tasks, sustained 's', breath flow was free flowing and relaxed. However, the therapist was unable to extend the cough into voicing and James began to inhibit the cough. Other initial attempts to facilitate voice also failed.

James seemed keen to talk and he volunteered significant information. His father had been in hospital for the last few months suffering a breakdown and had recently returned home. His brother Tom, who was a year younger, had severe mood swings. James explained that he and his brother were both having counselling at school. He also mentioned a much younger 4-year-old sister. Finally, James explained that he had changed school a year ago and had moved out of private education and away from his close friends. James painted a picture of being rather lonely and solitary at home and keen for some support and for a return of voice.

To normalise his situation and to reassure him, the most supportive approach for James was for the therapist to explain that voice loss does sometimes follow colds, that his voice would return and that voice therapy may help to speed this up. At the same time the therapist gave recognition of the stresses James was experiencing at home and gently explained that they would have played a part in his voice problem. James opted for some therapy.

The time the therapist then spent with James's mother was equally illuminating because amongst other things she explained more fully that her husband had been arrested from the home suddenly 10 months earlier and had been in prison. He had quite recently returned home and was unwell and not fit to stand trial. The family faced a lot of uncertainty about their future and had had to come to terms with a very reduced income and lifestyle. She also explained that she and the children would be leaving her husband and that the children were aware of this. James's mother also talked about both of the boys and their difficulties. She said that Tom had had severe behaviour difficulties for several years and that because his current behaviour was 'unbearable' he had recently been referred to a child psychiatrist. However, she felt that this was unproductive and that it served only to give Tom the attention that she felt he was seeking. In her view both children were getting some secondary gain from their behaviours and she mentioned a recent and unconnected emergency admission to hospital when James felt he was seriously ill and she believed that he was malingering or over-dramatising. The therapist gained the impression that she was only just coping with life herself and had limited patience for the boys' difficulties. Despite this she did see the damaging consequences of social isolation for James resulting from both his aphonia and spending his time alone in his bedroom.

The therapist gave James's mother a more direct explanation of psychogenic aphonia and reassured her that James's voice would return when he was happier in himself and more relaxed. Meanwhile the therapist offered to work with James and to visit the school in order to gain their cooperation and support for James.

Finally the therapist met with both James and his mother to explore the way forward. It was agreed that the therapist would visit the school that week and would talk to key members of staff and to the school counsellor and that James would attend for some voice therapy.

From this initial session it was not difficult to postulate the key aetiological factors of this psychogenic aphonia:

- James had experienced significant and sustained stress at home both prior to his father's arrest and since.
- He had witnessed the breakdown of his father and his brother's behaviour problems.
- He was aware of the struggle this situation created for his mother and of an uncertain future for himself.
- He had left the security of his long-term friends and had become quite alone.

Despite being aware of his father's arrest, the fact that he chose to talk about hospitalisation rather than imprisonment probably reflected his difficulty in coming to terms with this traumatic event. Finally, he did not describe any emotional support, and his mother's inability to empathise with her son probably reinforced his isolation and fear. Nevertheless his open communication of his emotional state, his keenness for support and the reports of some voicing were good prognostic indicators for voice and these and other indicators suggested that this was a Type 2 psychogenic voice disorder.

This case study also provides a good example of the choices the therapist has in explaining a psychogenic voice disorder. James could more easily accept an explanation of muscle tension dysphonia resulting from a throat infection and that the muscles needed some help to be programmed to work easily again. It felt important not to challenge this young lad who was struggling in his life, yet the therapist was able to begin to point out the link between his emotional stress and his muscles, even in the initial session. James's mother was already aware of the traumatic changes for the family and it was therefore appropriate to acknowledge the direct link that the stresses had in causing James's aphonia. In both cases reassurance and a positive plan for the future were signalled clearly by the therapist.

Therapy for James was given immediately and a resolution to normal voice was quick. The school visit played an important part in the therapy plan. The therapist met with the school's Special Educational Needs Co-ordinator (SENCO). Although the school had been aware of the home circumstances they had not understood that the aphonia was related to stress nor considered that James was struggling emotionally. The SENCO undertook to explain straightaway to the staff that the aphonia was not put on but was a reaction to stress; staff were asked to think about ego boosting for James but not to make him too special, i.e. to normalise. The therapist also suggested that the SENCO make contact with mum and invite her into the school so that the school could support the boys. The therapist met the school counsellor to explain the psychogenic nature of the voice loss and the therapist's involvement.

During the following two weeks James attended four sessions of voice therapy. In the first two sessions the therapist moved through a selection of facilitative techniques using firm modelling, voicing simultaneously to mask James's attempts and listening carefully for any success. Techniques used included:

- body release and jaw release
- cough, then extending and shaping this into vowels

- coordinated blowing and voicing on fricatives, 'zzz', adapted from Accent Method
- giggle and voice, adapted from Estill (Harris et al. 1998)
- creaky voice
- inhalation phonation.

Success varied and was limited but voice was heard unreliably on an extended cough, in creaky voice and on inhalation phonation. The therapist gave positive reinforcement, encouraged self-practice and gave permission for the voice to return as the muscles relaxed. In between these sessions James reported that it was becoming easier to produce voice, for example, when laughing, although it was inconsistent.

By the third session James had been able to produce voice more reliably on a laugh and a cough. Within that session voice was developed quite quickly from a vowel preceded by a firm glottal onset into extended vowels, polysyllables with rising and falling pitch 'oh oh', and into phrases, poetry, then conversation. All of this was achieved with firm modelling and some energetic exercise with big arm swings, stretches and jumps to emphasise the big vocalisations. Having established conversation with James, the therapist rang home and James spoke to his father, who was thrilled, so that James's voice could be generalised outside of the clinic. James discussed taking his voice outside of the clinic and said he would try to use it at school that afternoon. The therapist then rang school to let them know to expect James talking. The following week James was seen for the final session. His voice was normal and solid and he was very pleased to be able to talk.

The therapist now spoke with James about how he was coping. He had not been sleeping that week and he voiced his concerns for his father. He began to talk about how he felt his mother had cut herself off from him and that she was not there to listen to him. The therapist steered James to look at where his support lay and James responded that his grandparents listened to him and that at school he felt able to talk to his Head of Year and the counsellor.

Once again the therapist gave James positive reinforcement, reassuring him on his return of voice, offering ego-boosting on his success both with his voice and on his ability to talk to people who were there to lend support.

Following this session the therapist spoke with his Head of Year to suggest that he continues to help James with his self-confidence through ego-boosting in the form of positive feedback, praise, etc. When James failed to appear for his review appointment three weeks later, the therapist assumed that he no longer had a need for voice therapy. Telephone contact was made with his father two weeks after that and he reported that James's voice had been fine and that even despite getting tonsillitis he had not lost his voice.

CASE SUMMARY

This case study illustrates a Type 2 psychogenic aphonia and a resolution based primarily on symptomatic voice therapy. The case does highlight the importance of the psychosocial case history and suggests how this can be conducted with an adolescent and parent. Understanding the aetiology enabled the therapist to empathise effectively with this young patient, to recognise the value of confidence and ego-boosting for him and of helping him to access available support. It also shaped the therapist's treatment programme with regards to the liaison with the school, which was a key environment to offering ongoing support to this lad.

Predisposing factors

Personality was not explored, however he presented as someome who needed and enjoyed friendships and the support of others.

Precipitating factors

Stress and anxiety associated with the trauma of his father being arrested and impri-soned. Choosing to describe this as 'hospitalisation' rather than imprisonment empha-sised James's difficulty in openly expressing his anxieties and emotions about this trauma. His move from the security of his school and from close friends left him isolated and lonely, with no support and no one to confide in. He therefore dealt with the anxiety on his own through suppression.

The fact that James had a preceding URTI may have weakened the site (i.e. the throat) where his emotional conflict was somatised. This weakened resistance may have influenced the timing of the onset of the voice loss.

Perpetuating factors

He continued to witness the breakdown of his father and of the family at home. His mother's own distress meant that she was unable to effectively communicate with or support James. His isolation was therefore intensified, as he had no opportunity to express his suppressed emotions. Furthermore, James was aware of his mother's distress and, to some extent, was protecting her and this may have given rise to some conflict over his speaking out.

James's recent hospital admission, with an unrelated psychosomatic presentation further illustrated the stress that he was experiencing, his psychological tendency to somatise stress and possibly an attempt to gain attention and sympathy. However, this was not reciprocated by his mother – who was in fact irrirated and unsympathetic.

ANNE: TYPE 2 (COGNITIVE BEHAVIOURAL CONVERSION) APHONIA

PRESENTATION

Anne was referred to SLT by ENT with aphonia of acute onset. Fibreoptic examination had been traumatic for the patient but had shown a normal larynx. Her voice loss had commenced six weeks prior to her attending SLT and had followed a flu-type illness that had lasted approximately three weeks. Although in her mid-twenties, Anne attended her initial appointment with both her parents. Anne was invited into the therapy room alone but her mother requested she sit in during the appointment, 'to speak for her (Anne) as she can't make herself understood'. Anne accepted this arrangement with a shoulder shrug.

Anne had limited eye contact with the therapist during the case history and deferred most questions to her mother who in contrast to Anne's introversion, was forceful and direct in her approach to questioning, although dismissive of psychological questioning. It proved very difficult to extract a detailed social and personal history. The therapist felt that Anne and her mother were side-stepping questions around family and emotional issues. It was possible however to ascertain that Anne was an only child, who lived and worked with her parents as members of a religious organisation. Her social life seemed focused around the church and her parents. There appeared to be limited extended family and no identified friendships. Both Anne and her mother attributed her voice loss to her flu-type illness. There were no reports of previous episodes of dysphonia or voice loss.

Since her voice loss she had continued to go to work and carry out some of her secretarial duties but no longer used the phone or had contact with the public. She and her mother denied any significant life events and/or conflicts.

TREATMENT

The therapist felt troubled by Anne's considerable sense of sadness and withdrawal during the session. It was felt important to obtain some privacy for Anne, and the therapist therefore asked her mother to step out of the next part of the session while Anne worked through some exercises to re-establish her voice. Her mother agreed to this and waited in the waiting area with Anne's father.

The therapist worked through a series of tasks including cough-phonate, creaky phonation and shoulder shrug-phonate. Anne's approach to tasks was inhibited and childlike. She was giggly (no voice) and hesitant and needed initial coaxing to use eye contact with the therapist and perform the tasks. Voice was established and developed rapidly into speech through chanting. Her response to hearing her voice was to break down in tears as if heartbroken rather than relieved. The therapist sat quietly with Anne until she looked up and said, 'Please don't tell mum and dad.'

Further gentle questioning and reassurance by the therapist persisted with Anne crying although she denied any stressors or worries. She became very distressed again when the therapist asked her 'whether she was having any difficulties with anyone at home or in her family' but again felt unable to speak out. It was agreed with Anne that she should return the following week for a follow-up appointment where she could work further on her voice and further explore possible triggers for her dysphonia. Her parents were advised that the initial treatment session had been very encouraging and that a return of voice seemed highly likely.

Anne failed to attend her follow-up appointment. The therapist wrote directly to her inviting her to contact her to discuss treatment. Anne wrote back saying that her voice had returned and that she did not wish to attend for further appointments but she wanted to thank the therapist for helping her. Although nothing was specifically said the therapist was left feeling a sense of discomfort over this case. Anne's response to her return of voice was overwhelming. The family's approach to interview and Anne's own response to questioning left the therapist with a sense of sadness and concern for Anne's physical and mental wellbeing; however, without concrete evidence of emotional control/abuse, it was difficult to take these concerns further once the therapist's direct invitation to make contact was declined by Anne.

CASE SUMMARY

This case would seem to fit a Type 2 psychogenic voice disorder. The voice returned to normal quickly through the use of symptomatic voice therapy and yet this was clearly not the whole story. Although Anne was unable to express any inner conflict verbally, the therapist was given many clues that Anne was using suppression rather than repression as a coping mechanism. With hindsight the therapist believes the better approach would have been to explore the psychological factors in more detail and gain Anne's trust before accessing her voice and removing her defences.

SUE: TYPE 2 (COGNITIVE BEHAVIOURAL CONVERSION) DYSPHONIA

PRESENTATION

Sue was a 42-year-old senior bank clerk referred to speech and language therapy from the ENT department with a normal larynx and 'acute hoarseness'. At assessment she explained that she had become dysphonic suddenly six weeks earlier. Initially her voice had been persistently hoarse, but she reported occasional periods of normal voice more recently. Her voice was held in a high falsetto quality, she did not complain of soreness but felt tightness around her larynx and a 'frog' in the throat.

Sue had attributed her voice loss to laryngitis although she agreed with the therapist that she had not had an upper respiratory tract infection. Having taken a medical history and details of the voice loss the therapist broadened the case history to examine the areas described in Chapter 4, namely:

- identifying events and stresses in Sue's life over the preceding year and particularly immediately preceding the dysphonia;
- examining symptoms of stress, anxiety and physical tension;
- interpersonal relationships;
- her ability to express her views.

It was quickly evident that Sue had had a very traumatic year. Her husband had had an affair and had left her 10 months earlier, which she recalled as a 'horrendous' time.

She initially lost two-and-a-half stone in weight, experienced an anxiety state and had attempted an overdose three months later. She then had a period of counselling, which she had recently finished. She was unhappy in her job and she explained that she had transferred a lot of the anger towards her husband onto her boss, who she knew was having an affair, and this had caused a lot of difficulty in the work place. Her disabling dysphonia occurred at a time when she was particularly unhappy with her boss and when she was worrying about her future security.

She described her husband as 'a power freak' who continued to let himself into the house, taking some control of her life and would not let her go. Although she seemed to have made a lot of positive adjustments she was in a double bind. She did not want to lose her house but she also would like to move on. However, she was unable to move on or truly separate from her husband while she remained in the house. In fact, she was very angry at the prospect of losing her house. During this case history taking Sue's voice became increasingly more modal.

From this case history the therapist was able to recognise that this was a psychogenic voice disorder attributed to the significant life stresses and emotions that Sue was experiencing. She had made a lot of adjustments to her circumstances but was not yet able to make some final decisions. The decision to accept permanent separation and to lose her house was clearly painful. She continued to be angry both about her husband's betrayal and about the prospect of giving up her house. Nevertheless she expressed the view that she did not want her husband any more, that she did not want him to keep returning to the house and that she did need some financial security.

The therapist's tentative hypothesis was that the main inner conflict and stress was Sue's anger towards her husband combined with her relative powerlessness over this controlling man who continued to enter her home and who had financial control of her. This unexpressed conflict and stress had converted itself into the dysphonia.

During the assessment the therapist adopted some of the principles of CBT outlined in Chapter 3, namely:

- creating a sound therapeutic relationship, enabling the patient to trust and to feel understood;
- thinking holistically and systematically, particularly recognising the links in this case history between the life events, the interpersonal relationship and how these were shaping Sue's cognitions, emotions and physiological reactions (loss of weight, sleeplessness for example);
- active listening;
- reflecting back thoughtfully in a way that might help Sue to understand her difficulties;
- asking good questions;
- formulating a tentative hypothesis;
- and finally, providing the client with a clear review of the therapist's thoughts, findings and formulation.

The feedback given to Sue at the end of the session was based on reassurance and demystification of the problem. Sue was given a simple explanation of the link between stress and voice loss and, having discussed the stresses in her life so fully, it was easy for her to understand that these stresses might inevitably result in her voice disturbance. The therapist was deliberately neither challenging nor directive in the action that she felt might be best for Sue but through applying the CBT assessment principles Sue was given the opportunity to verbalise her current dilemma over her house and separation. The therapist strongly reassured Sue that her voice could return to normal quickly and based on the fact that the voice became almost normal during the session suggested they met in a few days to release the voice through a sequence of exercises. Since Sue was keen to get back to work as soon as she could, she was keen to take up this offer. The therapist also reflected on the many positive adjustments that Sue had made in her life and indeed on her openness and her insightfulness.

When Sue returned four days later she arrived in falsetto voice but reported two days of normal voice following the assessment. She had reflected a great deal on the assessment session and had arranged for a valuation of the house for the following week. She had begun to consider that moving house could have advantages, a view not expressed before. Sue said she realised that she was not quite ready to completely accept separation from her husband, although she could see many benefits if she did. Significantly she had arranged to meet her husband to talk about the valuation and the future and she had insisted that they meet on neutral territory at a place of her choosing. This more assertive behaviour did seem to suggest that Sue wanted to take charge rather than feel controlled.

The therapist was able to empathise and to reflect back to Sue on the difficult decisions that she was facing but also to help Sue to recognise that she was taking charge. She also reflected positively on many examples of good coping ability that Sue described and finally reinforced some of the examples where Sue had taken positive steps to do things to make herself feel better, (for example, redecorating some of the house in colours and furnishings of her choice and not of her husband's).

The therapist then guided Sue firmly through a sequence of voice exercises designed to release her high larynx setting and move her back to modal voice. The therapist worked with Sue standing in order to encourage an open, balanced body and to combine breath and voice release with open body gestures. The therapist gave Sue good modelling and initially vocalised with Sue in order to mask her first attempts and to minimise any embarrassment. The exercises included:

- hum
- hum through a descending glide
- firm expiratory 'hmm'
- 'hmm' on a descending glide
- intoned speech (in modal voice)
- glottal onset of vowels, polysyllables, words
- finally conversation.

Through this symptomatic voice therapy Sue achieved strong, normal voice and she was very pleased to have her voice restored.

A further appointment was made for a week later but Sue rang to cancel this appointment. However, when she phoned to cancel she explained that she had managed a full week at work and had maintained modal voice. She had also had the meeting with her husband and said she was clearer about her future. She did not volunteer more information but it was agreed that she was managing well and would be discharged.

CASE SUMMARY

This case study illustrates a Type 2 psychogenic voice disorder. The CBT assessment principles helped Sue to see the connections between her life events and her voice, to recognise that she had decisions to make about her future when she was ready to do so and perhaps to lead her to behave more assertively with her husband. From a psychological perspective we would say that she needed to overcome the anger and inhibition created by her husband's thoughtless and controlling behaviour, assert herself, express her feelings or 'find her voice' and make positive behavioural change. The case study also illustrates the important role that symptomatic voice therapy has and that a combined approach was rewarding for this client.

Schemas/personal beliefs

These were not fully assessed by the SLT; however, Sue apparently found it difficult to believe in the right to fully express anger towards her husband in order to assert herself or to set limits.

Predisposing factors

Husband's infidelity 10 months earlier led to acute stress and anxiety state.

Precipitating factors

Sue was unable to express her anger, her fears and her needs and was unable to prevent her husband from continuing to enter the house. She remained financially dependent on her husband for security of her home. Fear of losing her home increased her anger towards her husband.

Sue was unhappy at work. She projected her anger towards her husband onto her boss, this made their working relationship increasingly difficult.

Perpetuating factors

Sue's continuing feelings of powerlessness and anger towards her domineering husband. Unresolved work tensions.

SHARON: TYPE 2 (COGNITIVE BEHAVIOURAL CONVERSION) DYSPHONIA

PRESENTATION

Sharon presented as a tall, well-groomed and attractive woman in her mid-twenties. She was referred to one of the authors (PB) by her GP and presented with feelings of depression, having panic attacks, and symptoms of agoraphobia. At the first assessment she did not complain of any difficulties with her voice and none were noticeable during the interview. We have described her case in detail in a previous publication (Butcher et al. 1993) but it so perfectly illustrates a classical Type 2 picture that we feel it is worth repetition. Working with Sharon was also one of those rare, if not unique, occasions when a therapist has an opportunity to witness at first hand the emergence of Type 2 dysphonia while attempting to treat an individual's depressive-anxiety symptoms, loss of self-esteem and difficulty expressing views and feelings.

ASSESSMENT

Sharon appeared to have had a good relationship with her parents and elder brother and her early life was unremarkable. She left school to become a professional dancer but stopped dancing professionally when she became pregnant at the age of 21. Her long-term relationship with her boyfriend broke up at this stage and she found it difficult to return to professional dancing. Thus, she found herself forced to take a succession of less and less glamorous jobs. At the time of assessment she had a job collecting cash from slot machines in pubs and clubs.

Sharon described herself as someone who 'had to be better than the girl next door' and said that her loss of self-esteem and self-confidence began when she was no longer able to dance and had failed to make a career as a model. Her symptoms of anxiety and depression began after she lost one of her slightly more glamorous jobs working in the travel industry. For the past two years she had been in a relationship with a man called Kevin and they planned to marry in six months time. She expressed ambivalence about the idea of marriage. While there were very positive aspects to the relationship, she felt that Kevin was very controlling, gave her little opportunity to be herself or express what she wanted, and added that 'he treats me like a little girl.'

TREATMENT

The initial focus in the first three treatment sessions was on (1) stress management training, (2) improving both her communication and self-assertion with Kevin, and (3) increasing the rewards in Sharon and Kevin's relationship. However, at the fourth session Sharon had become dysphonic and could only speak in a hoarse, whispering voice. She described how the day before she lost her voice Kevin's mother had given her a bouquet to carry down the aisle that was not to her taste and, out of fear of offending her future mother-in-law, she said nothing about her feelings. To make matters worse, the following day she discovered that her dog had chewed up the bouquet and now Sharon felt this was a second thing she could not speak to Kevin's mother about. Within a short space of time and on the same day that her dog chewed up the bouquet, Sharon lost her voice. At this session Sharon also revealed that although she felt she had made some progress in being more frank about her feelings, she had many concerns about the forthcoming marriage that 'I haven't been able to say to Kevin.' In the light of this it was agreed that she would invite Kevin to the next session in the hope that, with therapeutic support, she would be able to be more open and honest with her partner.

At this next meeting, Kevin presented as having a particularly forceful personality with a strong tendency to take control of proceedings. Despite this controlling quality in Kevin's make-up, it was clear that the couple shared a great deal of warmth, affection and humour. As the session developed it became possible for the couple to discuss Sharon's inhibition in speaking her mind and to explore areas where they both had difficulty in communicating. One outcome that seemed important was that Kevin was able to admit that he tended to be bossy and blunt like his mother as well as poor at explaining himself and that there were occasions when things 'came out wrong'. Because the therapist was able to use the discussion to stress the value of improving both the communication and rewards in their relationship, the couple were able to use the last part of the session to set specific targets to make positive changes during the coming week.

Although invited to come to following meetings, Kevin did not attend again. However, Sharon reported at the next session that he had made more effort with communicating and had set limits at work in order to meet her request of spending more time together in the evenings. Moreover, she described how, for the first time, she was able to confront him about his habitual untidiness and expectation that she would tidy up after him.

At following meetings Sharon continued to report successes in self-disclosure and expressing her concerns. Notable among these successes was talking with Kevin about playing a role in disciplining her daughter, expressing her fears that the marriage would give his mother greater influence in her life, and confronting Kevin with his immature attitude to financial management. This progress grew steadily out of analysing each difficulty in the therapeutic hour, then preparing or practising homework that might help her make the changes she targeted. For example, after some preparation in a session on how to speak to Kevin about their financial arrangements, she felt she was able to put this into action very successfully. On reflection, however, she then realised that she had not said all she wanted to say and, on her own volition, went back to the subject and even threatened to call off the marriage unless he stopped taking her for granted and began to 'show he is a partner'.

Sharon was clearly growing in self-confidence and assertiveness and in the following weeks had to deal with two new dilemmas involving speaking her mind. First, a friend of Kevin's mother revealed to Sharon that her future mother-in-law had confided that she didn't believe Sharon's dog had destroyed the bouquet and had implied that this was just Sharon's excuse because she did not like it. Second, although Kevin had continued to be tidier and less bossy, he was still not being 'a partner' when it came to financial matters. Although at this time she did not find the courage or find a way to confront Kevin's mother concerning the bouquet, she did speak to Kevin about helping more with the finances. In addition, because she was determined not to let anything major spoil her wedding day, she made a special and successful trip to visit Kevin's sister so that she could speak about a misunderstanding which had caused a great deal of tension between both parties for some months.

Shortly afterwards, on the actual day of the wedding, Sharon experienced a noticeable improvement in her voice. For three months her voice had been a just audible, frequently hoarse, whisper. Now she described a sensation as though her voice was 'going to burst out at any minute'. Then, after three-to-four weeks of fluctuating voice quality and periods of 'croakiness', her voice returned to normal. As we summed up in the previous discussion of this case:

> She said this occurred at a time when, having taken the step into marriage, she was feeling more confident about her relationship with Kevin, of expressing her views and of showing her independence. In particular, she felt that she was able to be a woman in her own right and that Kevin had accepted and adapted well to this. Thus, she said, she felt relieved to find her worst fears unfounded. Because of her new found confidence in herself, she had also been able to be more outspoken and to confront her employer, who had been making unreasonable work demands, and other staff members who had been treating her badly. As a consequence of speaking her mind in this situation, she was much happier at work and this stress greatly diminished. There had been a significant decline in her depressive/anxiety symptoms and, shortly after, she was discharged from treatment.
>
> Butcher et al. 1993, p. 106.

CASE SUMMARY

This case documents the onset of PVD in a woman coping with stressful life and identity changes associated with failing to achieve her ambition to be a dancer or model. She initially presented in the psychology department with symptoms of depression, anxiety, panic attacks, and lowered self-esteem. Her dysphonia emerged in the context of being in conflict with a man she was shortly to marry, who was highly controlling and treated her 'like a little girl'. The specific trigger was being unable to say what she genuinely felt about the gift of a bridal bouquet and its destruction by her dog. Successful resolution of the dysphonia appeared related to employing a variety of cognitive behavioural strategies – detailed analysis of problem areas, communication and assertiveness training, target setting and behavioural experiments – to help her take control and verbalise her feelings.

Schemas/personal beliefs/rules of living

I have to be better than the girl next door.

Predisposing factors

Loss of self-esteem; a 'driven' personality; being infantilised in her relationship with her partner; not being heard or allowed to express her views.

Precipitating factors

Not feeling able to say what she felt about her bridal bouquet.

Perpetuating factors

Continuing to be inhibited in expressing feelings about the bouquet, Kevin's controlling nature, his discipline of her daughter, his untidiness and his poor financial management; life change associated with the transition into marriage.

KATIE: TYPE 2 (COGNITIVE BEHAVIOURAL CONVERSION) DYSPHONIC TEENAGER

PRESENTATION

Katie, a 17-year-old, presented with a four-week history of dysphonia commencing after an episode of flu. She attended the appointment with her mother who sat in on the session. Katie reported being initially aphonic and after several days had developed a strained whisper. Since then she had heard her true voice on a number of occasions, i.e. once when talking to her godmother, for a brief period after her ENT appointment and several times when laughing. She reported no laryngeal discomfort but felt she had to 'push to make (my) voice work'. Katie also had a six-month history of breathing difficulties with a sensation of tightness in her chest. Medical tests for this had been negative and Katie told the therapist she thought it may be asthma although she was not taking any medication. Katie then told the therapist that her older brother had died from an asthma attack 10 years previously. Her ENT examination also ruled out any organic cause for her dysphonia.

Katie presented as bright and animated and close to her mother who also attended the appointment. Katie reported being worried that her voice problem might interfere with her oral A level exams in a few months time. Her dysphonia, she said was also preventing her from participating in her pleasure pursuits of singing in the church choir and drama.

Katie's voice was severely dysphonic and characterised by breathiness, a raised pitch and low volume. Palpation of the laryngeal and head and neck muscles indicated a high held larynx, significant tongue base tension and laryngeal tension and tenderness. Voice production was characterised by general body tension, raised shoulders and upper chest breathing. She had a strong cough.

TREATMENT

As Katie was clearly keen to re-establish a normal voice and had been encouraged already by brief episodes of normal voice, the therapist decided to defer a detailed psychological history until she had probed Katie's voicing potential within the first session. Normal voice was established in the first session by encouraging a lower laryngeal posture and vocal fold approximation using cough-phonate, yawn-sigh, shoulder shrug-phonate and chanting techniques. This focus was preceded by laryngeal manipulation.

Voice was developed into spontaneous speech in this first session although Katie's breathing remained clavicular and her general presentation was tense. The association between voice loss and tension and stress was discussed with Katie and she was asked to consider any aspects that may have been causing her worry or stress around the time or leading up to the episode of her voice loss. Katie described herself as a worrier and agreed to return for a follow-up appointment to explore psychological factors further. The therapist contacted Katie by telephone five days later and was encouraged to hear that she had maintained normal voice and had returned to normal activities in singing and drama.

At her follow-up appointment three weeks later, the psychological issues that may have contributed to the development of her voice loss were explored with Katie. Her mother agreed to sit outside for this session. Katie started by describing herself as a worrier and admitted in particular to having had exam worries. The therapist explored the basis for Katie's concerns. Katie expressed her fear that she could not match up to her brother's achievements at the same age. He had died 10 years previously, at the age of 18, and had excelled academically. She felt both her parents, and in particular her mother, felt disappointed in her academic abilities and did not rate her artistic talents although she knew they loved her. Katie's personal report suggested that her mother was still grieving the loss of her son and that she frequently cried and talked about him to Katie. His death had been sudden and unexpected and the family had attended some counselling sessions soon after. Katie had very little memory of these sessions. She denied any fear of dying suddenly herself and talked rationally about the cause of and events leading up to her brother's death. She admitted however, to feeling the need to protect her mother from further hurt by disappointing her in any way. She had not discussed her feelings with her mother but had confided a little in her godmother who lived abroad.

Katie was able to see that her symptoms of voice loss and breathing difficulties could be linked to her feelings of conflict and anxiety and the burden of responsibility in trying to protect her mother. Katie agreed to her mother joining the remainder of the session and disclosed her feelings to her mother with facilitation by the therapist. They were both tearful during the session and open and honest about their feelings for each other and Katie's brother. It was agreed that Katie would benefit from psychological therapy, the focus being to further explore her thoughts and feelings, focus on changing her dysfunctional thoughts about her self-worth, teach her stress management techniques and assertiveness skills. She was referred via her GP for CBT. Her mother also decided to access bereavement counselling services.

CASE SUMMARY

Personal schema

I am not as good as my brother; I am inadequate; I must not disappoint my mother.

Stressful life experiences

Sudden loss of older brother 10 years previously; maternal grief.

Predisposing factors

Worrier, anxious.

Precipitating factors

Loss of brother; approaching age at which brother died; approaching exams; not as academically able as brother; fear of hurting mother/fear of maternal rejection.

Perpetuating factors

Fear of expressing feelings; continued belief that 'I am not good enough'; muscular tension.

LYDIA: TYPE 3 (PSYCHOGENIC-HABITUATED) APHONIC TEENAGER

PRESENTATION

Lydia, a 15-year-old, was referred to Speech and Language Therapy with a six-month history of aphonia. ENT examination had confirmed normal vocal fold mobility and a normal laryngeal structure. Two weeks prior to the onset of her aphonia she reported having had an accident at school in a chemistry class in which she had inhaled chlorine fumes. She reported feeling a burning sensation in her throat that went on to last a week although without any change in voice. She saw the school nurse and GP and stayed off school for a week. She then caught a viral infection, with a cough, sore throat and dysphonia, developing to aphonia over a period of a week. Since then she reported being consistently aphonic, hearing some voice on only a few occasions, e.g. when coughing, laughing and hiccupping.

She attended the appointment with her mother. Together they reported feeling that her problem had been caused by the inhalation of chlorine. There was no suggestion that they were taking further action with the school over the accident and Lydia discussed her frustration at not being able to communicate well with her friends and family.

She was aphonic throughout the assessment phase of the session. Palpation of her head and neck indicated a high, held larynx with tension and tenderness. Voice production was accompanied by generalised body tension, upper chest breathing and tense shoulders. She produced a strong glottic cough.

TREATMENT

Voice therapy techniques were explored in the first session with the aim of establishing normal voice. Cough-phonate, yawn-sigh, shoulder shrug-phonate and laryngeal manipulation were used to initiate vocalisation on sustained sounds, progressing quickly towards chanting on phrases. Live biofeedback of vocal fold activity was provided at this stage using the electrolaryngograph as Lydia developed her chant into spoken phrases. Out of task Lydia remained aphonic.

She was delighted to have heard her voice and the suggestion was made that she should expect her voice to return over the next few days. The remainder of the session was spent exploring psychological factors that might explain the development and maintenance of her voice problem. An association between voice loss, muscle tension and stress was explained to Lydia, who seemed very receptive to this concept. Although initially reticent, Lydia did start to talk about her anxiety around the time of her accident in chemistry and with gentle questioning admitted that she had felt partly responsible as she and her friend had been dismissive of some of the instructions given by her teacher during the experiment. She had initially feared that she had burned her throat and that she would be permanently damaged. She felt her mother had been very supportive in arranging for Lydia to see a specialist but suggested that at the time her mother's anxiety had made her worry more that 'things were bad'. She had not felt able to tell her mother what had really happened as she felt this might result in her friend getting into trouble as well and a possible suspension that might affect her chances of doing well in her exams. Lydia had the opportunity to talk through the accident with her school teachers. Her mother had also attended this meeting, which she had found supportive. Lydia volunteered that she felt the issues around the accident were now sorted out and that she understood that there was no permanent harm to her throat. She did not express any ongoing anger or upset over this episode and her mother said she felt the school had acted appropriately in trying to sort out why it had happened. Lydia had remained off school for the initial two weeks after the accident but had since then attended school and was preparing for mock exams. She was no longer worried that her exam chances were threatened.

Her family was close, although she had no contact with her father. Lydia described a loving relationship with her grandparents and cousins and her younger siblings. She described herself as a 'worrier' and as 'getting stressed easily'. She liked to be 'quiet' and enjoyed the company of a small group of friends 'whom I am very close to'. She spent her social time with these friends and exploring internet chat rooms. During the session it was not possible to identify any perpetuating factors associated with the maintenance of her dysphonia but Lydia was asked to give this further thought before her next appointment.

Later that day, Lydia telephoned to say that her voice had returned fully in conversation and she expressed her delight and said she had telephoned her mother straight away and that they had been in tears together. The therapist suggested that her voice should now remain constant and suggested she continue to carry out her yawn-sigh exercises until a review appointment in five days time.

At this review appointment, Lydia reported no voice difficulties. Her breathing pattern remained clavicular and she continued to present with some generalised body tension. She was taught systematic relaxation and how to centre her breathing pattern. She had identified no ongoing stressors in her life aside from her mock exams, which she felt were going fine. We agreed that the antecedent to her difficulties was likely to have been the chemical inhalation, associated both with acute anxiety and probable inflammatory response creating a 'soft spot' at the level of the larynx that was further sensitised by the viral infection a few weeks later. Lydia's early fears/anxieties about the accident and her conflict over speaking out had gradually dissipated with the positive support of her mother and meetings with the school and ENT doctors. No ongoing psychological factors were identified and it was agreed that Lydia's voice difficulty had been maintained due to a habituated muscle tension response. It is likely that her personality characteristics had predisposed her to worry and that this had contributed to the development and maintenance of her symptoms. It was recommended she regularly use relaxation techniques to manage these tendencies. No further follow-up was recommended. In this case Lydia's voice problem was clearly associated with a traumatic event but with no dissociation (for further discussion see Chapter 1 p. 19).

CASE SUMMARY

This case provides an example of a Type 3 (psychogenic-habituated) aphonic patient. Although there was an obvious traumatic event clearly associated with the throat, her dysphonia did not develop into aphonia for several weeks afterwards. This may have been due to psychological processes alone but could also have developed as a result of hyperfunctional voice use. Psychological screening suggested there were no unresolved issues for the patient, some six months after the accident and onset of her problems. We would suggest that Lydia felt early emotional conflict relating to fears of permanent damage, which may have been suppressed and a conflict over speaking out about her own responsibility for what happened. Lydia achieved a quick recovery of voice through the use of symptomatic voice therapy techniques. Psychosocial questioning around the three Ps at the time of assessment, helped to raise her awareness of a tendency to worry and thus heightened her receptiveness to relaxation techniques as a mechanism for dealing with symptoms of stress.

Personal schema

I am a quiet person; I am liked and loved; I need to do well.

Traumatic life experiences

Chemical inhalation at school.

Predisposing factors

Worrier, anxious, introverted.

Precipitating factors

Chemical inhalation at school; viral infection; conflict over speaking out about own responsibility for accident; fear of permanent damage to her throat.

Perpetuating factors

Habituated muscle tension behaviours.

JANE: MUSCLE MISUSE DYSPHONIA

PRESENTATION

Jane was a 51-year-old preschool teacher referred to psychology for an assessment following speech therapy for moderate–severe dysphonia. The referral letter stated the following:

> She initially presented to speech therapy with moderate–severe dysphonia, although ENT examination revealed no abnormality. Her dysphonia appeared to be the result of increased laryngeal tension, which we have now remedied by teaching her how to balance the resonance and tension between her larynx and the rest of her vocal tract. She reports that she now has a normal voice more often than not, and when her voice does deteriorate she is now generally able to return to normal within seconds through simple exercises to refocus her resonance. It would appear that the dysphonia is related to stress – as she reports her voice goes when she gets uptight and at times she is unable to get it back, even through the exercises she has been prescribed, if she is particularly stressed.

PSYCHOLOGICAL ASSESSMENT

At interview Jane described herself as happily married for 25 years. There were no personal or financial stresses and no unusual tensions in her relations with her husband and their two grown up daughters who were now in their twenties. She was very positive about her course of voice therapy and the improvement in her voice but her voice had deteriorated on recently restarting work.

She described how prior to starting work the previous week she was quite nervous and she felt 'the nerves' had affected her voice. However, she had plans in place for an assistant to take over if her voice deteriorated and at these times she planned to go to a spare room to do her voice exercises. Psychologically, Jane admitted to having a tendency to worry and to being conscientious, but the assessment did not suggest that these characteristics fell too far outside the normal range. This was supported by the HADS, which was normal for depression and showed only mild levels of anxiety.

There were no indications that her voice problem was related to internal conflicts with conflicts over speaking out, or external pressures in the form of major relationship difficulties or unresolved personal conflicts or concerns. From a psychological point of view her voice problem could be explained by her conscientiousness and a related tendency to be over-persistent or not to give up too easily. There was evidence that there were some areas that she avoided due to her voice disorder but she seemed to be overcoming these. For example, she had been avoiding answering the telephone but had been doing this in recent weeks. Similarly, although she had been avoiding social situations because of the strain on her voice, she described a plan to gradually develop her social life once she was settled in at work. At interview she was very aware of the need to not overuse or to rest her voice and to continue her voice exercises.

TREATMENT

At assessment Jane's progress was such that there did not seem a major focus for psychological treatment or for additional behavioural targets and a review was arranged at three weeks. At this review she reported that she had reduced her hours at work because her voice had deteriorated. In retrospect she felt it had been a mistake to go straight back to full-time work because she was using her voice all the time and the breaks she had were usually not enough to rest her voice. However, she had continued to do her voice exercises regularly and she felt that resting her voice continued to be helpful. Interestingly, she reported feeling guilty about taking time off to rest her voice while at work and suggested that her over-conscientiousness played an important part in her voice deterioration. Although this was focused on in the session there were no behavioural targets set as Jane had already arranged to work half-time over the following month and it was agreed to meet again at the end of this time to review how helpful she found this strategy.

At the third meeting Jane reported that although her voice had been very good in the week of half term, working a shorter day from 8:45 in the morning to 1:30 in the afternoon had not been enough to get the voice back to normal. After discussion Jane agreed to set four targets for the following month: 1. Speak with her manager and arrange either to work shorter hours or to have more time to rest her voice while at work. 2. Speak to colleagues and explain that she needs to rest her voice more frequently. 3. Initiate voice rest *at the very first sign* of voice deterioration. 4. Keep record sheets of voice problems and rest times. Jane cancelled her next appointment and when seen at five weeks it was clear that there had been problems fully carrying through with her targets. She had spoken to her manager and had reduced her working day by a further half hour. During the first week she had four days with perfect voice but then developed flu, which caused her to lose her voice completely and from which it took a long time to recover. In fact, she felt so low and tearful after the flu that on consulting her GP she was prescribed a course of antidepressants. At this meeting it was planned that she used the following two weeks of half term to fully recover and that on return to work she would implement what remained of the targets from the previous session. Jane failed to attend her next appointment four weeks later and was re-booked for the following week at which she reported that her voice had been fine since her two weeks off. She also reported being much better at monitoring her voice and that she had been working full-time for nearly three weeks. She had continued the antidepressant medication as she felt it reduced feelings of panic but emphasised that the improvement in her voice was associated with a number of behavioural changes. This included being better at monitoring voice change, being more disciplined with not straining her voice (for example, not reading so long to the children and instead of shouting to call them in from play she would let others do it) and regularly doing voice exercises in a small storage room when she needed more support for the voice. At this point she was encouraged to maintain her new behaviours and a review was arranged at six weeks. At this follow-up Jane had been working full-time for two months and reported that, overall, her voice had been 'very good'. She estimated that her voice still deteriorated about once a week but associated this with a pattern of occasional overuse. Each time, however, the voice loss was short-lived and always responds to rest. Importantly, from a cognitive perspective, Jane described how the occasional voice problem no longer caused her to panic and assume she had 'gone back to square one'. She was now able to stay relaxed, trust that the problem was due to strain and that it would resolve with voice rest. Because of her progress in managing her dysphonia Jane was discharged from treatment and did not contact the department for further help.

CASE SUMMARY

In presenting with laryngeal tension that quickly responds to voice therapy and voice care, Jane is typical of cases with muscle misuse voice disorder. By quickly relapsing, she is also fairly typical of those patients who find it hard to set limits, reduce stresses or make the necessary healthy lifestyle changes. It is common with these cases that voice therapy is rarely enough to prevent relapse, even when, to some extent, the patient keeps up the recommended voice exercises and voice care. As shown in this case, it is always important to consider strategies that target unhealthy patterns of thinking and behaving. In this case, her primary problems were (1) being unable to reduce the strain on her voice due to her perfectionistic tendencies or difficulty admitting that she needed help; (2) a failure to monitor her voice consistently while reading or raising the volume; and (3) not taking appropriate action as a result of the monitoring (e.g. use voice conservation).

Schemas/personal beliefs/rules of living

I must be seen to be hard working; I must do things well/perfectly; I must not be seen by others to be weak; I should not ask for help.

Predisposing factors

Perfectionistic traits; conscientiousness; vocal misuse. Although there were some personality traits that encouraged muscle tension behaviours there were no significant emotional or psychosocial issues.

Precipitating factors

Vocal strain through raising her voice to be heard and through long periods reading out loud to the children.

Perpetuating factors

Continued voice misuse; failure to monitor voice and note deterioration early; not reducing hours or taking time out to rest voice or asking for help from colleagues on noticing early signs of voice loss; panic caused by belief that voice loss meant she had 'gone back to square one'.

REFERENCES

Abramson LY, Seligman MEP and Teasdale, JD (1978) Learned helplessness in humans: Critique and reformulation. *Journal of Abnormal Psychology*, **87**, 49–74.

American Psychiatric Association (2000) *Diagnostic and Statistical Manual of Mental Health Disorders*, 4th edn, Text Revision. Washington, DC, American Psychiatric Association.

Andersson K and Schalen L (1998) Etiology and treatment of psychogenic voice disorder: Results of a follow-up study of thirty patients. *Journal of Voice*, **12** (1), 96–106.

Arntz A (1994) Treatment of borderline personality disorder. A challenge for cognitive-behaviour therapy. *Behaviour Research and Therapy.* **32** *(4)*, 419–30.

Aronson AE (1990a) *Clinical Voice Disorders*, 3rd edn. New York: Thieme.

Aronson AE (1990b) Importance of the psychological interview in the diagnosis and treatment of 'functional' voice disorders. *Journal of Voice*, **4** (4), 287–9.

Aronson AE, Peterson HW, and Litin EM (1966) Psychiatric symptomatology in functional dysphonia and aphonia. *Journal of Speech and Hearing Disorders*, **XXXI** (2), 115–27.

Austin C (1997) The identification of psychological and social processes involved in psychogenic voice disorder. University of East London. Dissertation.

Azrin NH and Besalel VA (1981) An operant reinforcement method of treating depression. *Journal of Behaviour Therapy and Experimental Psychiatry*, **12** (2), 145–51.

Baker J (1998) Psychogenic dysphonia: Peeling back the layers. *Journal of Voice*, **12** (4), 527–35.

Baker J (2002) Psychogenic voice disorders – heroes or hysterics? A brief overview with questions and discussion. *Logopedics Phoniatrics Vocology*, **27**, 84–91.

Baker J (2003) Psychogenic voice disorders and traumatic stress experience: A discussion paper with two case reports. *Journal of Voice*, **17** (3), 308–18.

Bandura A (1989) Perceived self-efficacy in the exercise of personal agency. *The Psychologist*, **2** (10), 411–24.

Barskey AJ (1989) Somatoform disorders. In (Eds), *Comprehensive Textbook of Psychiatry*. HI Kaplan and BJ Sadock London: Williams and Wilkins.

Bateman A and Fonagy P (1999) Effectiveness of partial hospitalization in the treatment of borderline personality disorder: A randomized control trail. *American Journal of Psychiatry*, **156** (10), 1563–9.

Beck AT and Emery G (1985) *Anxiety Disorders and Phobias: A Cognitive Perspective*. New York: Basic Books.

Beck AT, Freeman A and Associates (1990) *Cognitive Therapy of Personality Disorders*. London: Guilford Press.

Beck AT and Steer RA (1987) *Beck Depression Inventory*. Sidcup: The Psychological Corporation.

Beck AT and Steer RA (1990) *Beck Anxiety Inventory*. Sidcup: The Psychological Corporation.

Bennett-Levy J (2003) Mechanisms of change in cognitive therapy: The case of automatic thought records and behavioural experiments. *Behavioural and Cognitive Psychotherapy*, **31**, 261–77.

Boone DR (1977) *The Voice and Voice Therapy*, 2nd edn. Englewood Cliffs, NJ: Prentice Hall.

Boone D and McFarlane S (1993) A critical view of the yawn-sigh as a voice therapy technique. *Journal of Voice*, **7** (1), 75–80.
Boone D and McFarlane S (2000) *The Voice and Voice Therapy*. 6th edn. Needham Heights, MA Allyn and Bacon.
Brodnitz FS (1969) Functional Aphonia. *Journal of Otolaryngology*, **78**, 1244–53.
Burns DD (1980) *Feeling Good*. New York: Morrow.
Butcher P (1983) The treatment of childhood-rooted separation anxiety in an adult. *Journal of Behaviour Therapy and Experimental Psychiatry*, **14** (1), 61–5.
Butcher P (1984) Existential-behaviour therapy: A possible paradigm? *British Journal of Medical Psychology*, **57**, 265–74.
Butcher P (1994) Psychogenic voice loss: Psychological features and treatment. *Clinical Psychology Forum*, **69**, 2–4.
Butcher P (1995) Psychological processes in psychogenic voice disorder. *European Journal of Disorders of Communication*, **30**, 467–74.
Butcher P (2000) *Managing Stress: A practical guide*. Audio-tape and booklet, available from baglady2k @ hotmail.com.
Butcher P and Cavalli L (1998) Fran: Understanding and Treating Psychogenic Dysphonia from a Cognitive-Behavioural Perspective. *Wanting to Talk* (ed. D Syder). London: Whurr.
Butcher P and Elias A (1983) Cognitive-behavioural therapy with dysphonic patients: An exploratory investigation. *The College of Speech Therapists Journal*, **377**, 1–3.
Butcher P and Elias A (1994) Psychological features of voice disorder and treatment strategies. *You Are Your Voice*. British Voice Association Conference, London: Regents College.
Butcher P, Elias A and Raven R (1993) *Psychogenic Voice Disorders and Cognitive-behaviour Therapy*. London: Whurr.
Butcher P, Elias A, Raven R, Yeatman J and Littlejohns D (1987) Psychogenic voice disorder unresponsive to speech therapy: Psychological characteristics and cognitive-behaviour therapy. *British Journal of Disorders of Communication*, **22**, 81–92.
Chadwick P and Birchwood M (1994) The omnipotence of voices: A cognitive approach to auditory hallucinations. *British Journal of Psychiatry*, **164**, 190–201.
Clark DM (1986) A cognitive approach to panic. *Behaviour Research and Therapy*, **24**, 461–70.
Clark DM (1996) Panic disorder: From theory to therapy. In *Frontiers of Cognitive Therapy* (ed. PM Salkovskis). New York:Guilford.
Colton RH and Casper JK (1996) *Understanding Voice Problems: A physiological perspective for diagnosis and treatment*, 2nd edn. Baltimore, MD: Williams and Wilkins.
Daniilidou P (2006) *Voice Therapy and Cognitive Behavioural Therapy in Functional Dysphonia*. 9th Newcastle Voice Conference. Newcastle, UK.
Davison GC and Neale JM (1978) *Abnormal Psychology: An experimental clinical approach*. Chichester: John Wiley & Sons, Ltd.
Davison GC and Neale JM (1982) *Abnormal Psychology: An experimental clinical approach*. Chichester: John Wiley & Sons, Ltd.
Deary IJ, Scott S, Wilson IM, White A, Mackenzie K and Wilson JA (1997) Personality and psychological distress in dysphonia. *British Journal of Health Psychology*, **2**, 333–41.
Dryden W and Ellis A (1988) Rational-emotive therapy. In *Handbook of Cognitive-behavioural therapies* (ed. KS Dobson). London: Hutchinson.
Ehlers A and Clark DM (2000) A cognitive model of posttraumatic stress disorder. *Behaviour Research and Therapy*, **38**, 319–45.

Eifert GH and Forsyth JP (2005) *Acceptance and Commitment Therapy for Anxiety Disorders: A Practitioner's Guide to Using Mindfulness and Values-Based Behaviour Change Strategies.* Oakland CA: New Harbinger Publications.

Elias A, Raven R, Littlejohns D and Butcher P (1989) Speech therapy for psychogenic voice disorder: A survey of current practice and training. *British Journal of Disorders of Communication,* **24**, 61–76.

Falloon IRH (1985) *Family Management of Schizophrenia: A Controlled Study of Clinical, Social, Family and Economic Benefits.* Baltimore, MD: John Hopkins University Press.

Fourcin A (1986) Electrolarynogographic assessment of vocal fold function. *Journal of Phonetics,* **14**, 435–42.

Freeman M (1991) When is a voice disorder psychogenic? Some considerations for diagnosis and management. In *Voice Disorders and their Management* (ed. M Fawcus), London: Chapman Hall.

Freud S (1962) The aetiology of hysteria. In *Complete Psychological Works.* London: Hogarth Press.

Friedl W, Friedrich G and Egger J (1990) Personality and coping with stress in patients suffering from functional dysphonia. *Folia Phoniatrica* **42**, 13–20.

Froeshels E (1948) *Twentieth Century Voice Correction.* New York: Physiological Library.

Garety PA and Freeman D (1999) Cognitive approaches to delusions: A critical review of theories and evidence. *British Journal of Clinical Psychology,* **38**, 113–54.

Gath D and Goeting NLM (1990) *Panic: Symptom or disorder. Current approaches.* Southampton: Duphar Medical Publications.

Gelder MG (1990) Psychological treatment for depressive disorder. *British Medical Journal,* **300**, (28 April), 1087–154.

Gerritsma EJ (1991) An investigation into some personality characteristics of patients with psychogenic aphonia and dysphonia. *Folia Phoniatrica* **43** (1) 13–20.

Greene M and Mathieson L (1989) *The Voice and Its Disorders,* 5th edn. London: Whurr.

Grey N, Young K and Holmes E (2002) Cognitive restructuring within reliving: A treatment for peritraumatic emotional 'hotspots' in posttraumatic stress disorder. *Behavioural and Cognitive Psychotherapy,* **30**, 37–56.

Guze SB and Brown OL (1962) Psychiatric disease and functional dysphonia and aphonia. *Archives of Otolaryngology,* **76**, 84–7.

Hackmann A (1998) Cognitive therapy with panic and agoraphobia: Working with complex cases. In *Treating Complex Cases: The cognitive behavioural approach* (eds N Tarrier, A Wells and G Haddock). Chichester: Wiley.

Hammarberg B (1987) Pitch and quality characteristics of mutational voice disorders before and after therapy. *Folia Phoniatrica,* **39**, 204–16.

Harris T, Harris S, Rubin J and Howard D (1998) *The Voice Clinic Handbook.* London: Whurr.

Harris T and Lieberman J (1993) The Cricothyroid mechanism, its relation to vocal fatigue and vocal dysfunction. *Voice,* **2**, 89–96.

Hayes SC, Strosahl KD and Wilson KG (2003) *Acceptance and Commitment Therapy: An Experiential Approach to Behaviour Change.* London: Guilford Press.

Haywood A and Simmons R (1982) Relaxation groups with dysphonic patients. *The Bulletin of the College of Speech Therapists,* 359.

Hirano M (1981) *Clinical Examination of the Voice.* Vienna: Springer.

Holland SJ (1997) Obsessive-compulsive disorder. In *Practicing Cognitive Therapy: A Guide to Interventions* (ed. R Leahy). London: Aronson.

House AO and Andrews HB (1987) The psychiatric and social characteristics of patients with functional dysphonia. *Journal of Psychosomatic Research*, **31** (4), 483–90.

House AO and Andrews HB (1988) Life events and difficulties preceding the onset of functional dysphonia. *Journal of Psychosomatic Research*, **32** (3), 311–19.

Huxley A (1964) *Island.* Harmondsworth: Penguin.

Jacobson E (1938) *Progressive Relaxation.* Chicago, IL: University of Chicago Press.

Janet P (1920) *The Major Symptoms of Hysteria.* New York: Hafner.

Juniper D (1978) *How to Lift Your Depression.* London: Open Books.

Kinzl J, Biebl W and Rauchegger H (1988) Functional aphonia. A conversion symptom as defensive mechanism against anxiety. *Psychotherapy and Psychosomatics*, **49**, 31–6.

Koschkee D and Rammage L (1997) *Voice Care in the Medical Setting.* San Diego, CA: Singular.

Koufman JA and Blalock PD (1982) Classification and approach to patients with functional disorders. *Annals of Otology, Rhinology and Laryngology*, **91**, 372–7.

Kovac M, Rush AJ, Beck AT and Hollon SD (1981) Depressed outpatients treated with cognitive therapy or pharmacotherapy: One-year follow-up. *Archives of General Psychiatry*, **38**, 33–9.

Lam DH, Jones SH, Hayward P and Bright JA (1999) *Cognitive Therapy for Bipolar Disorder: A therapist's guide to concepts, method and practice.* Chichester: Wiley.

Laver JD (1980) *The Phonetic Description of Voice Quality.* Edinburgh: Edinburgh University Press.

Linehan MM (1993) *Cognitive-behavioural Treatment of Borderline Personality Disorder.* New York: Guilford Press.

Linklater K (1976) *Freeing the Natural Voice.* New York: Drama Book Publishers.

Lockhart MS, Paton F and Pearson L (1997) Targets and Timescales: a study of dysphonia using objective assessment. *Logopaedics Phoniatrics Vocology*, **22**, 15–24.

Lombard E (1911) Le signe de l'elevation de la voix. *Annales Maladies Oreilles Larynx Nez Pharynx*, **37**, 101–19.

Martin S and Lockhart M (2000) *Working with Voice Disorders.* Bicester, Oxon: Winslow Press Ltd.

Mathieson L (2001) *Greene and Mathieson's The Voice and its Disorders*, 6th edn. London: Whurr.

Meichenbaum D and Cameron R (1973) Training schizophrenics to talk to themselves: A means of developing attentional controls. *Behaviour Therapy*, **4**, 515–34.

Meichenbaum D and Genest M (1982) Cognitive behaviour modification: An integration of cognitive and behavioural methods. In *Helping People Change* (eds FH Kanfer and AP Goldstein). New York: Pergamon.

Millar A, Deary IJ, Wilson JA and Mackenzie K (1999) Is an organic/functional distinction psychologically meaningful in patients with dysphonia? *Journal of Psychosomatic Research*, **46** (6), 497–505.

Morrison MD and Rammage LA (1993) Muscle misuse voice disorders: Description and classification. *Acta Otolaryngology* **113**, 428–34.

Nordby, VJ and Hall, CS (1974) *A Guide to Psychologists and Their Concepts.* San Francisco, CA: Freeman.

Padesky CA (1994) Schema change processes in cognitive therapy. *Clinical Psychology and Psychotherapy*, **1** (5), 267–78.

Padesky CA (2002) *Cognitive Therapy Unplugged.* www.cognitiveworkshops.com

Perley MJ and Guze SB (1962) Hysteria – the stability and usefulness of clinical criteria. *New World Journal of Medicine*, **266**, 421–6.

Powell T (2000) *The Mental Health Handbook*. Bicester: Speechmark Publishing.

Rachman SJ and Hodgson RJ (1980) *Obsessions and Compulsions*. Englewood Cliffs, NJ: Prentice-Hall.

Raine R, Haines A and Sensky T (2002) Systematic review of mental health interventions for patients with common somatic symptoms: Can research evidence from secondary care be extrapolated to primary care? *British Medical Journal*, **325**, 1082–93.

Rattenbury H, Carding PN and Finn P (2004) Evaluating the effectiveness and efficiency of voice therapy using transnasal flexible laryngoscopy: A randomised trial. *Journal of Voice*, **18**, 522–33.

Rogers CR (1961) *On Becoming a Person*. Boston, MA: Houghton Mifflin.

Rotter JB (1966) Generalised expectancies for internal versus external control of reinforcement. *Psychological Monograph*, **80** (1), 1–28.

Roy N, McGory J, Tasko SM, Bless DM and Ford CN (1997) Psychological correlates of functional dysphonia: an investigation using the Minnesota Multiphasic Personality Inventory. *Journal of Voice*, **11**, 443–51.

Rush AJ, Beck AT, Kovacs M and Hollon SD (1977) Comparative efficacy of cognitive therapy and pharmacotherapy in the treatment of depressed outpatients. *Cognitive Therapy and Research*, **1**, 17–37.

Ryle, A (1990) *Cognitive Analytic Therapy: Active participation in change*. Chichester: John Wiley & Sons, Ltd.

Salkovskis PM (1989) Obsessions and compulsions. In *Cognitive Therapy in Clinical Practice: An Illustrative Casebook* (eds J Scott, JMG Williams and AT Beck). London: Routledge.

Salkovskis PM (1996) The cognitive approach to anxiety: Threat beliefs, safety-seeking behaviours and the special case of health anxiety and obsessions. In *Frontiers of Cognitive Therapy* (ed. PM Salkovskis). New York: Guilford.

Salkovskis PM and Hackmann A (1997) Agoraphobia. In *Phobias – A Handbook of Theory, Research and Treatment* (ed. GCI Davey). Chichester: John Wiley & Sons Ltd.

Scott S, Deary IJ, Mackenzie K and Wilson JA (1997) Functional dysphonia: A role for psychologists? *Psychology, Health and Medicine*, **2** (2), 169–80.

Segal ZV, Williams JMG and Teasdale JD (2002) *Mindfulness-based Cognitive Therapy for Depression*. London: Guilford Press.

Seligman MEP (1975) *Learned Helplessness: On Depression, Development and Death*. San Francisco, CA: Freeman.

Shafran R (1999) Obsessive compulsive disorder. *The Psychologist*, **12** (12), 588–91.

Shewell C (2000) The voice of experience. *Bulletin of The Royal College of Speech and Language Therapists*, **November**.

Sisti M (1997) Hypochondriasis. In *Practicing Cognitive Therapy: A guide to interventions* (ed. R. Leahy). London: Aronson.

Smucker MR (1997) Post-traumatic stress disorder. In *Practicing Cognitive Therapy: A Guide to interventions* (ed. R. Leahy). London: Aronson.

Snaith RP, Constantopoulos AA, Jardine MY and McGuffin P (1978) A clinical scale for the self-assessment of irrationality. *British Journal of Psychiatry*, **132**, 164–71.

Teasdale JD (1988) Cognitive vulnerability to persistent depression. *Cognition and Emotion*, **2**, 247–74.

Teasdale JD, Segal ZV and Williams JMG (1995) How does cognitive therapy prevent depressive relapse and why should attentional control (mindfulness) training help? *Behaviour Research and Therapy*, **33**, 25–39.

Teasdale JD, Segal ZV, Williams JMG, Ridgeway VA, Soulsby JM and Lau MA (2000) Prevention of relapse/recurrence in major depression by mindfulness-based cognitive therapy. *Journal of Consulting and Clinical Psychology*, **68** (4), 615–23.

Thyme-Frokjaer K and Frokjaer-Jensen B (2001) *The Accent Method. A rational voice therapy in theory and practice*. UK: Speechmark.

Tucker HM (ed.) (1987) *The Larynx*. New York: Thieme.

van der Kolk B, McFarlane AC and Weisarth L (1996) *Traumatic Stress*. New York: Guildford Press.

Warwick HMC and Salkovskis PM (1989) Hypochondriasis. In *Cognitive Therapy in Clinical Practice: An illustrative casebook* (eds J Scott, JMG Williams and AT Beck). London: Routledge.

White A, Deary IJ and Wilson JA (1997) Psychiatric disturbance and personality traits in dysphonic patients. *European Journal of Disorders of Communication*, **32** (3), 307–14.

Williams JMG (1984) Cognitive-behaviour therapy for depression: Problems and perspectives. *British Journal of Psychiatry*, **145**, 254–62.

Williams JMG, Watts FN, Macleod C and Mathews A (1988) *Cognitive Psychology and Emotional Disorders*. Chichester: John Wiley & Sons Ltd.

Wolpe J (1958) *Psychotherapy by Reciprocal Inhibition*. Stanford, CA: Stanford University Press.

Yalom ID (1980) *Existential Psychotherapy*. New York: Basic Books.

Yanagisawa E, Citardi M and Estill J (1996) Videoendoscopic analysis of laryngeal function during laughter. *Annals of Otology, Rhinology and Laryngology*, **105** (7), 545–9.

Yates AJ (1970) *Behaviour Therapy*. London: John Wiley & Sons Ltd.

Young JE and Brown G (2003) *Schema Questionnaire*. Published by Cognitive Therapy Centre of New York, 36 West 44th St, Suite 1007, New York, NY 10036, USA. *www.schematherapy.com*

Zigmond AS and Snaith RP (1983) The hospital anxiety and depression scale. *Acta Psychiatrica Scandinavica*, **67**, 361–70.

INDEX

Printed in the United States
By Bookmasters